The Brain Injury Workbook

The Brain Injury Workbook

Exercises for Cognitive Rehabilitation

Trevor Powell & Kit Malia

Headway
the brain injury association

Speechmark

www.speechmark.net

A note on the text
The logos that appear on page 85 are the registered trademarks of the respective companies.

Published by
Speechmark Publishing Ltd, 70 Alston Drive, Bradwell Abbey, Milton Keynes MK13 9HG, United Kingdom
Tel: +44 (0)1908 326944 Fax: +44 (0)1908 326960
www.speechmark.net
Headway – the brain injury association, 4 King Edward Court, King Edward Street, Nottingham NG1 1EW, United Kingdom
www.headway.org.uk

First published 2003
Reprinted 2004, 2005, 2006, 2008 (twice), 2010 (twice)

002-5079/Printed in the United Kingdom by CMP (UK) Limited

British Library Cataloguing in Publication Data

Powell, Trevor J., 1955–
The brain injury workbook : exercises for cognitive rehabilitation
1. Brain damage – Patients – Rehabilitation 2. Group counseling
I. Title II. Malia, Kit III. Headway (Organisation)
617.4'81'0443

ISBN: 978 0 86388 318 7

Contents

PART III: EMOTIONAL ADJUSTMENT

Preface

Since the early 1990s, cognitive rehabilitation has developed from a 'fashionable accessory' into an indispensable therapeutic approach for any centre that professes to provide good comprehensive rehabilitation for brain-injured people. This is an exciting, young and developing field that has a great deal to offer to people with brain injury. In my experience over the last 16 years, clients and their families have expressed the same complaint – not having enough information about, and practical help with, their cognitive problems. These problems persist for many years after the initial injury, and in many cases seem to get worse. This book will provide much needed resources to help people working in this field, to help clients with brain injury to maximise their abilities. I am therefore very happy to have been involved with the production and 'road testing' of the materials in this book.

Please let us know how you get on with the exercises and information sheets, so that we can continue to develop useful and appropriate materials.

Kit Malia
Cognitive Rehabilitation Therapist

Acknowledgements

This book has evolved over the last fifteen years through working in groups, and individually, with people struggling to come to terms with life after a brain injury. I would like to thank all those people whose experiences have shaped this book. This specifically includes all those in the Monday Headway group and the Thursday Battle Hospital group.

I would also like to thank a long list of clinicians that I have worked with over the years. A special thanks to Tanja Gillham, my colleague at Battle Hospital. Thanks also to Anne Jeavons, Rob Stevens, Marigold Hayes, Huw Williams, Bob Lamperd, Shelagh Grier, Maggie Cooper, Annabelle Glover and Kit Malia. Gratitude also to the team at Headway Thames Valley, the West Berks Clinical Psychology Department and those at Battle Hospital Rehabilitation Unit in Reading. My appreciation also goes out to anybody else whose ideas I have borrowed, copied or plagiarized.

Trevor Powell
October 2003

Introduction

This book has evolved gradually over the last 15 years, during which time I have run outpatient therapy groups and courses for people with an acquired brain injury – mainly head injury. These groups and courses have been part psychotherapeutic, part educational and run on a semi–structured format. This book is a collection of exercises, games and information sheets used in these groups. Such groups are enormously popular with clients as they provide the opportunity to bring together people with similar problems, to provide support and to share and learn from each other. Research suggests that 'bringing people together' into small groups or a therapeutic milieu is an important component in rehabilitation (Ben-Yishay *et al*, 1985). Over and above that 'coming together and sharing', there are five main therapeutic aspects to this approach in these groups:

1 **Focused stimulation:** One of the Headway coordinators used to call out before the start of a group, 'Come on get those little grey cells working.' There is increasing evidence from new research that particular kinds of mental exercises activate or 'light up' particular parts of the brain, and the more the brain is worked the more efficient the neural pathways become (Goldberg, 2001). As Robertson (2000) so succinctly put it, 'cells that fire together wire together'. Others talk about 're-embroidering the damaged neural networks'. We are beginning to understand that the brain might have more of the qualities of a muscle than originally thought, and that therefore it needs exercising and training.

2 **Learning compensatory coping strategies:** If you have a disability you need to find a way around it, or a way of coping. Just as with a physical disability you may have to walk with a stick, with a cognitive problem you have to find a way of compensating or coping. You might do something simple, like using a diary, or you might adopt an internal strategy, like using visual images to remember. This approach is largely based on the early work of clinicians such as Barbara Wilson (1987), who was one of the first people to write about 'Memory Training Groups'. There are psychological approaches to managing all sorts of problems, from improving your memory, concentration or executive skills, to managing your anger, stress levels or fatigue.

3 **Acquiring insight and awareness:** Lack of insight and awareness is a major problem after brain injury, particularly after head injury. It is difficult to be objective about yourself at the best of times, and even more so after a brain injury. You gradually come to realise exactly what sort of residual difficulties you have – rather like the mist lifting off the top of a mountain. George Prigatano (1999)

talks about psychotherapy after brain injury as being a gradual process of helping the client to identify their problems, comparing it to 'slowly turning the lights on in a dark room full of bear traps'. This process may take years, and still be only partial. Research has shown that lack of insight is one of the major obstacles to rehabilitation, returning to work and adjustment. All the exercises in this book are aimed at improving insight – helping you to see yourself more clearly and accurately, and to feel more in control and confident.

4 **Emotional adjustment:** A brain injury is a life-changing event, but at first you may not be aware of that. Gradually as insight improves you will begin to alter your expectations and accept your limitations. There will be difficult challenges and emotional upheaval, but out of this will come adjustment, and then some form of accommodation and acceptance. You accept that life has changed to some extent, and that there is no going back. It is rather like the process of bereavement, or mourning the loss of a loved one. With adjustment comes the ability to talk about what has happened; recognise what has changed, and move on with life. The final section of the book contains exercises that focus on adjustment.

5 **Improve self-efficacy of feeling more 'in control':** After a brain injury most people feel out of control and are desperate for knowledge and advice to help them feel more in control. These exercises and information sheets are to help people understand what is going on – what their problems are – to develop a few coping strategies and to have something mentally stimulating to do, so that they feel more in control. Hopefully this enhances feelings of self-effectiveness and empowerment – 'I am doing something about my problems.' This in turn improves motivation and builds confidence, which improves ability.

What is in this book?

This book is in six sections, with discussion sheets, questionnaires, quiz sheets and exercises for each. The first section is a group of general information sheets about brain injury. In my experience, clients and their families are always eager to learn and understand about what has happened to them. The second section is on memory; the third on thinking skills, and the fourth on executive skills. These are the major areas of cognitive impairment, and each section has information sheets, questionnaires, quizzes and exercises. The questionnaires are not standardised, and there have been no extensive validity tests. They are meant to be a stimulus for discussion and comparison. The different sections of the book have a certain amount of overlap, and the 'thinking skills' section is something of a ragbag of cognitive skills that do not fit easily into memory and executive skills. The fifth section of the book is on improving insight, and the sixth and largest section is on emotional adjustment. Again, there is obvious overlap in these areas.

Who should use this book?

This book is designed to be used in a number of different ways. It is based on material that I created to use in groups, and is therefore intended primarily as a resource for therapists working with brain-injured people in groups. It is a resource book or 'cookbook' where exercises or handout sheets may be photocopied and used therapeutically. However, all the exercises can be used by a therapist with clients on an individual basis. In addition, a person with a brain injury could work through the book on their own: clients or a family member often ask, 'Is there anything I can do to improve memory or thinking skills?' Finally carers, family members, and staff – for example at the Headway Day Centre – may use the book to provide stimulating activities for a brain-injured person.

The limitations of a cookbook

This cookbook approach might be seen as dangerous in the wrong hands. There is a risk: first, in timing, and second, in sensitivity and appropriateness. After a brain injury, you go through various different phases and stages, where different kinds of rehabilitation activity might be most appropriate. For example, the sheets on adjustment are not really suitable for a client within the first few months of their injury, because they are spontaneously improving all the time and do not really know what they need to adjust to. However, some of the sheets on thinking skills might be very appropriate. Similarly, there are many different types of brain injury: some people will have good executive skills and poor memories, and vice versa. It is generally accepted that people with severe memory problems and impaired executive skills are not very good at using internal memory strategies, whereas those with mild to moderate memory impairment and relatively intact executive skills do benefit. Many people with a brain injury do not like being thought of as having a disability; others are quite happy to accept this description. This needs to be handled sensitively, so the exercise sheets should be selected appropriately and tailored to individual needs.

Running groups and courses

Size

It is difficult to be prescriptive about the size of a group. I have run two types of groups over the years. The large open group at the Headway Centre may contain 20 people. The people often have severe disabilities and so the group has to move quickly. I also run a smaller, more intimate group with seven to nine members, for people with higher abilities. In the smaller group, the focus might well involve emotional adjustment, returning to work, or coping with other responsibilities; in the larger group, the emphasis might be more on stimulation, and learning coping strategies.

Length of time

The length of a session is important, but again there is no hard and fast rule. The Headway group runs for an hour, and certainly that is the maximum in terms of concentration, tolerance and fatigue thresholds for most of the members. The smaller group runs for one and a quarter hours. I have run groups where we have had a coffee break in the middle, after about 50 minutes. The only rule is to be aware of issues of fatigue, limited concentration span and tolerance levels, and not to overdo it.

Group membership

The vast majority of people in my groups have been people with a head injury. However, younger people who have had a stroke – particularly a subarachnoid haemorrhage – or people who have had a tumour removed, hypoxic brain injury, neurotoxic poisoning, or an infection such as encephalitis, might often benefit from taking part in a group.

Format

Over the years I have developed a typical format for my groups, which combines a mixture of structured activity and an opportunity to talk about how things are going. Typically, I start the group with 'a round', where each individual tells the group something about themselves. In the small group, individuals often tell about one positive and one negative thing that have happened in the last week. Everybody else in the group then has to link the positive and negative item with the person and remember it at the end of the group by creating a visualisation, or a picture in their mind. This kind of exercise combines all therapeutic aspects; offering an opportunity to practise memory strategies, providing stimulation, offers an opportunity to share with others and helps with insight and adjustment. After that, we might do a structured thinking skills exercise, a memory skills exercise, or an executive skills exercise. I then usually do an exercise that looks at some aspect of awareness or adjustment, where individuals can discuss a particular aspect of life after brain injury – this is the main part of the session. Because clients have cognitive impairment and reduced insight, it seems important to structure these discussion topics, and not to just expect such issues to come out spontaneously, as would happen in a normal psychotherapy group.

The poem on page xiii is written by a group member which seems to capture something of the essence of being in these groups and the material in this book.

I am not sure how this book will be received by other professionals, colleagues, carers and users, but at the very least it will be a useful way of structuring and ordering all the activities that I have used with people over the years. I hope it will be the beginning of a compilation that can be added to and refined over the years.

Trevor Powell
Consultant Clinical Neuropsychologist

References

Ben-Yishay Y *et al*, 1985, 'Neuropsychological Rehabilitation: Quest for a holistic approach', *Seminars in Neurology* 5(3), pp252–9.

Goldberg E, 2001, *The Executive Brain*, Oxford University Press, New York.

Robertson I, 1999, *Mind Sculpture*, Bantam Books, New York.

Prigatano G, 1999, *Principles of Neuropsychological Rehabilitation*, Oxford University Press, New York.

Wilson B, 1987, *Rehabilitation of Memory*, Guilford Press, New York.

What I gain from the group

The group takes me as I am.
They accept me, as they did not know me before.
So, I can relax completely, no need to be defensive.
They do not compare my behaviour, speech and attitudes with pre-accident.
If occasionally I get weepy and upset, it is handled without a fuss, but there is a feeling of understanding, because they have been there.
The worksheets are very, very useful because they help me where I need help.
They hit the spot and raise issues that I might not have thought about.
I feel myself becoming more aware and growing as a person.
The size is good, neither too small nor very big.
Everyone has space if they want it.
I enjoy the surprise of each session.
It's not boring and we always have a few laughs.

Jill

PART I

Education about Brain Injury

Education about Brain Injury

INFORMATION SHEETS

Information about traumatic brain injury

In the UK, one million people per year attend hospital with some form of head injury – 80 per cent are not admitted. About 270 people per 100,000 of the population are admitted to hospital with a head injury every year. Approximately 20 of these are severe head injuries, and the rest are either moderate or mild head injuries.

Causes of head injury

Road traffic accidents	50 per cent
Domestic and industrial falls	20–25 per cent
Sports and recreational injuries	10–15 per cent
Assaults	10 per cent

People who are most likely to have a head injury

- Males are three times more likely than females
- Most at risk are young males between the ages of 15 and 30 *(five times more likely)*
- People over 65 years are also more at risk
- People under the influence of alcohol
- People with a 'risk-taking' personality
- People who have had a previous head injury

The term 'silent epidemic' has been used to describe the increasing number of people who survive head injury. This is due to a combination of the increased speed of life in general, creating more injuries, and advances in medical technology saving more lives. It is estimated that 90 per cent of people with severe head injuries who survive today would have died 30 years ago.

In the USA 5.3 million people – more than 2 per cent of the population – live with a disability as a result of a brain injury. Less than 2 per cent of those have significant physical disabilities.

1 Why are more people today surviving head injury?
2 Who is most likely to have a head injury?

How relevant did you find this sheet? Very ☐ Slightly ☐ Not very ☐

What happens in a head injury?

In the majority of head injuries, the brain is accelerated and decelerated within the skull. Imagine what happens if you shake up a soft blancmange in a hard box – it shears, tears, and cracks. The injury is in two parts – primary and secondary injury.

Primary damage

(a) *Diffuse axonal injury.* At the moment of impact, the brain may strain or tear, and the microscopic nerve fibres, connections and axonal sheaths are stretched and ruptured.

(b) *Bruising (contusion).* Most common where the frontal and temporal lobes of the brain crash into the hard, bony ridges of the inside of the skull.

(c) *Primary bleeding and blood clots (haemorrhage and haematoma).* If an artery or other blood vessel tears and a blood clot forms, this may pressurise or squash the brain.

Secondary damage

(a) *Brain swelling (oedema).* The brain may swell, which reduces the flow of blood and oxygen to the cells of the brain and raises intercranial pressure.

(b) *Infections.* If the skull is fractured, germs may infect the brain.

(c) *Breathing problems (anoxia).* If there are injuries to other parts of the body, such as the heart or lungs, breathing difficulties may reduce the flow of oxygen in the blood to the brain.

(d) *Secondary bleeding.* A slow bleed may be detected only later (subdural, extradural, or intracerebral haematoma).

(e) *Cellular changes.* A cascade of biochemical events occur, including the release of various toxic neurotransmitters – glutamate, calcium and free radicals – which can lead to cell death.

1 What are the primary mechanisms of damage?
2 What secondary damage can occur?

How relevant did you find this sheet? Very ☐ Slightly ☐ Not very ☐

Measuring the severity of a head injury

The majority of head injuries are closed: the skull is not fractured, but the brain is accelerated and decelerated within the confines of the skull. These are different from open or penetrating head injuries, which might be the result of a gunshot wound, for example.

There are two major measures of how severe a head injury is:

(a) *Loss of consciousness.* This is measured by examining the client's ability to respond to a series of graded responses to external stimuli. These responses include responding to pain, opening and moving eyes to speech, and responding verbally to questions about orientation. A scale, called the Glasgow Coma Scale, measures these responses on a scale of 15 points, which measure depth of coma or consciousness. The lower the score out of 15, the more severe the head injury. A score of 13–15 indicates a mild or minor head injury.

(b) *Post-traumatic amnesia (PTA).* This is the time between the injury, and the regaining of day-to-day memory and an awareness of such information as time, date and surroundings. An approximate measure of PTA is to recall the first clear continuous memories you had after your injury. How long after the injury was it? A period of PTA of less than one hour indicates a mild head injury. A period of PTA of between one hour and 24 hours suggests a moderate head injury. PTA of over 24 hours suggests a severe head injury, and PTA of over seven days indicates a very severe head injury. The longer the period of PTA and the lower the Glasgow Coma Scale score, the more severe the injury and the more likely there are to be long term or permanent difficulties. These two measures are the best predictors of outcome.

1 What is the difference between a closed and open head injury?
2 How do you assess severity of head injury?

How relevant did you find this sheet? Very ☐ Slightly ☐ Not very ☐

Common consequences of brain injury

Physical

- ➤ Paresis – paralysis, inability to move part of the body; reduced mobility
- ➤ Ataxia – poor motor coordination; tremor
- ➤ Sensory loss – loss of sensational feeling
- ➤ Hearing impairment or tinnitus
- ➤ Visual difficulties – diplopia, blurred vision
- ➤ Loss of sense of smell and taste
- ➤ Balance problems – dizziness
- ➤ Headaches
- ➤ Fatigue – less stamina; tire more easily, need more sleep
- ➤ Epilepsy
- ➤ Sexual arousal

Cognition

- ➤ Executive skills impairment – poor planning, organising, initiation, poor problem solving and multi-tasking
- ➤ Memory impairment – poor short-term memory; problems with new learning
- ➤ Speed of information processing – slowed
- ➤ Attentional deficits – problems with sustained, divided, and switching attention
- ➤ Perceptual/visuo-spatial problems
- ➤ Language difficulties – understanding (receiving) or expressing (speaking)
- ➤ Loss of insight and awareness of changes and deficits

Emotion and behaviour

- ➤ Lowered tolerance of frustration – temper outbursts, easily angered
- ➤ Rapid mood swings – more moody and unstable
- ➤ Emotional lability – crying or laughing more easily
- ➤ Emotional flattening – reduced emotional sensitivity or tone (blunting)
- ➤ Apathy – reduced motivation and drive, little get up and go; reduced initiative
- ➤ Disinhibition – impulsiveness, saying what comes to mind; poor social judgement
- ➤ Anxiety, depressed mood, obsessionality – inflexibility

> What do you think are your five most serious problems after your brain injury?

How relevant did you find this sheet? Very ☐ Slightly ☐ Not very ☐

Areas of the brain and their function

The brain weighs about 3 lbs (1 kg), looks like two halves of a walnut, and has the consistency of blancmange.

Right and left hemisphere. The left hemisphere controls movement and sensation on the right-hand side of the body, and vice versa. For most people, the left hemisphere is important for language skills and the right is more important for spatial and non-verbal skills.

Frontal lobes. Located just behind the forehead. The chief executive or conductor of the rest of the brain. Important for all the skills that make us unique from other species, such as planning, organising, problem-solving, initiation, multitasking and other executive skills. Also important for control of personality, temperament, mood, emotions and speech.

Temporal lobes. Located just above the ears. Important for memory, hearing and understanding speech.

Parietal lobes. Located behind the ears, towards the back of the head. Important for spatial judgement, integrating sensory information, reading, writing and drawing.

Occipital lobes. Located at the back of the head. Important for vision, object recognition and identifying colour.

Cerebellum. Located below the occipital lobes at the back of the head. Important for coordination, fine motor movement, balance, walking and speech articulation.

Brain stem. This connects the brain to the spinal cord. Important for autonomic activities, such as alertness, breathing and swallowing.

Diencephalon and limbic structures. This is the ancient brain – a group of subcortical structures in the heart of the brain, involved with primitive emotions and drives. It includes the pea-sized hypothalamus (responsible for internal states, such as body temperature, appetite, arousal and sleep-waking); the amygdala (involved with emotions such as anger and fear), and the hippocampus (involved with memory).

1 What area of the brain is most important for executive skills, such as organising and planning, and why might this be larger in humans than in animals?
2 If you feel clumsier, poorly coordinated and have poor eye-hand dexterity, which part of the brain might have been injured?

How relevant did you find this sheet? Very ☐ Slightly ☐ Not very ☐

Cross-section of the brain

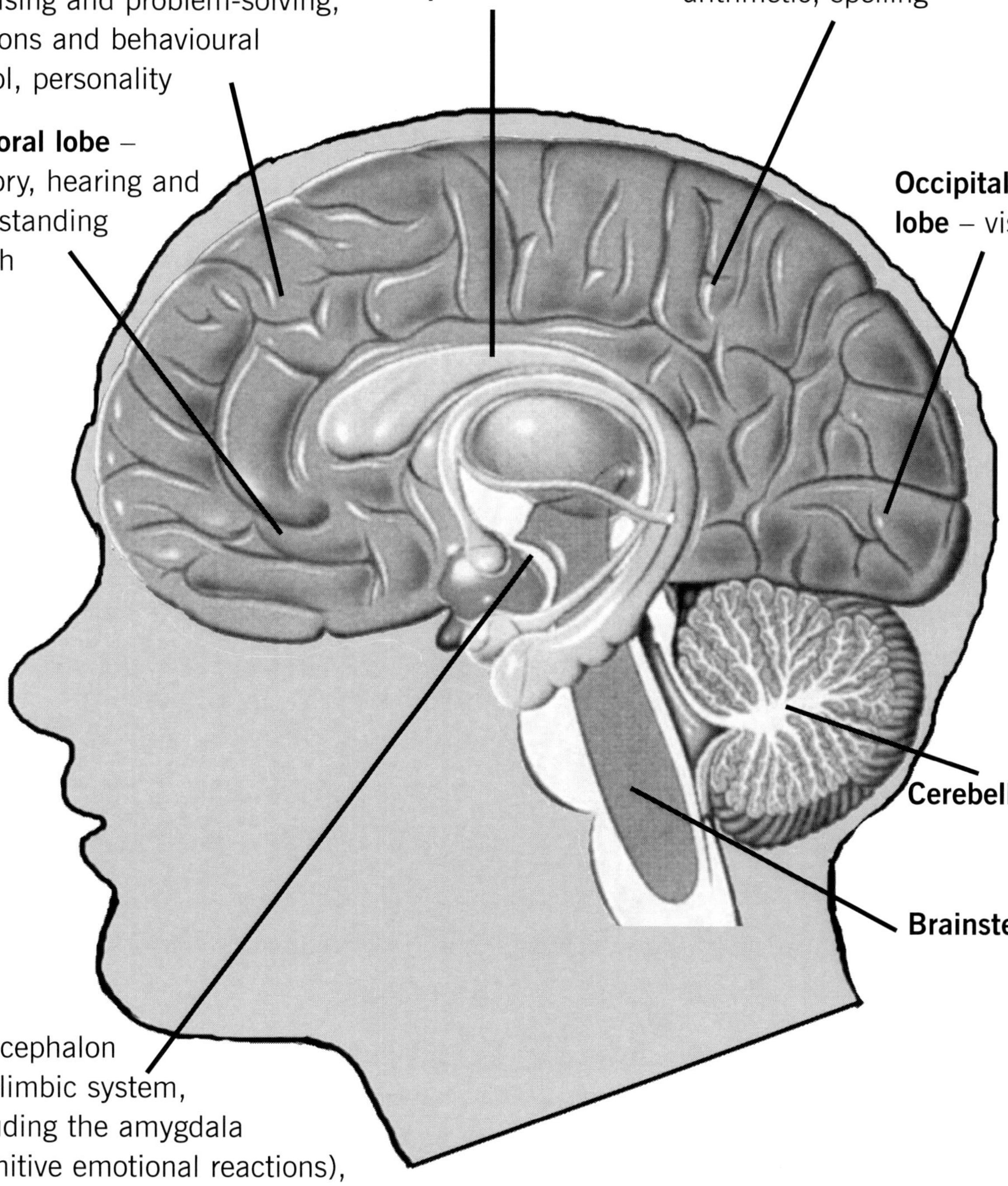

How relevant did you find this sheet? Very ☐ Slightly ☐ Not very ☐

Other major types of acquired brain injury

Acquired brain injury is a term that refers to any brain injury that is not congenital (there at birth), or is not degenerative (an illness that has a progressive decline). The following are some other conditions that can produce an acquired brain injury:

Strokes. When we say that someone has had a stroke, we are describing what has happened when the blood supply to some part of the brain is suddenly stopped, which leads to the death of that section of the brain. This is usually due to two main causes. First, the blockage of an artery carrying blood to the brain by a blood clot or 'infarct'. Second, a bleed or haemorrhage, either within the brain (intracerebral haemorrhage) or between the two delicate layers of membrane covering the surface of the brain (subarachnoid haemorrhage).

The incidence of stroke is approximately 200 per 100,000 of the population per year. Approximately one-third of the people who have a stroke die; one-third make a complete recovery, and one-third are left with some disability. Only 25 per cent of people who have a stroke and are left with disability are under the age of 65 years. 50–80 per cent of people who have a stroke have early paralysis on one side of their body. A stroke in the right side of the brain affects the left side of the body.

Neurotoxic disorders. These include neurotoxicity caused by alcoholism, carbon monoxide poisoning, or poisoning by solvents, metals, drugs, pesticides, or other neurotoxins.

Infections, such as meningitis and encephalitis. A viral infection can cause inflammation to the brain, which leads to swelling, and this pressure causes damage. Incident rate of approximately 30 per 100,000.

Hypoxia. Lack of oxygen to the brain. This often happens after a heart attack or coma caused by another illness, such as diabetes.

Cerebral tumours. The tumour itself may cause brain injury, or the neurosurgery or radiotherapy to remove the tumour may cause brain injury. Incidence rate of five per 100,000.

1 What happens when someone has a stroke?
2 Identify three types of illness that can cause brain injury.

How relevant did you find this sheet? Very ☐ Slightly ☐ Not very ☐

Self-assessment

1 What type of brain injury did you suffer?

___

2 What was the severity of your injury?

Lowest Glasgow Coma Scale score:

___

Length of post-traumatic amnesia:

___

3 What particular area of your brain was injured?

___

4 What are the results of any MRI or CT scans available?

___

5 My main physical problems are:

___

___

6 My main cognitive problems are:

___

___

7 My main emotional/behavioural problems are:

___

___

___

How relevant did you find this sheet? Very ☐ Slightly ☐ Not very ☐

PART II

Cognitive Rehabilitation

Memory

INFORMATION SHEETS

MEMORY EXERCISES

Memory questionnaire

Name ______________________ Date ______________

Read each of the statements, and mark the box that best describes your behaviour at present. It might be helpful to ask somebody who knows you well to complete the questionnaire and fill in the independent scorer column.

Scoring Agree = 2 Partially agree = 1 Disagree = 0

Question	**Score**					
	Self-score			Independent scorer		
	Agree	Partially agree	Disagree	Agree	Partially agree	Disagree
1 I often forget where I have put things in the house.						
2 I sometimes find a television story or the plot of a book difficult to follow.						
3 I often forget words, or find they are on the tip of my tongue and cannot quite find them.						
4 I often forget things, and have to go back for them.						
5 I sometimes forget things that I did the day before.						
6 I forget to do things that I have planned to do.						
7 I can tell somebody a story or joke that I have told before, or ask the same question twice.						
8 I sometimes forget to tell people important messages.						
9 I find it difficult learning a new skill (eg, working a computer, a game, a new gadget), or remembering a sequence of instructions.						
10 I sometimes fail to recognise places, or people's faces, that I have seen before and should be familiar with.						
TOTAL SCORE						

INTERPRETATION

Self-score

8–20: This suggests that you may have a poor memory, and may benefit from using compensatory strategies.

Discrepancy between self-score and independent score

5–20: This suggests that you may not be fully aware of your memory problem, or you are denying it.

How relevant did you find this sheet? Very ☐ Slightly ☐ Not very ☐

Understanding memory

Memory involves a number of different skills and stages, and can be likened to a sophisticated music system in which cassettes and CDs are recorded and stored, and then retrieved from storage and replayed when required. The first stage of memory is recording, which involves attending to and encoding the information perceived (selecting the cassettes or CDs and the tracks or sounds to record). The second stage involves storage of that information (placing the recorded cassette or CD somewhere safe). The third stage involves retrieving the information (identifying the correct cassette or CD, then putting it in the machine and playing it).

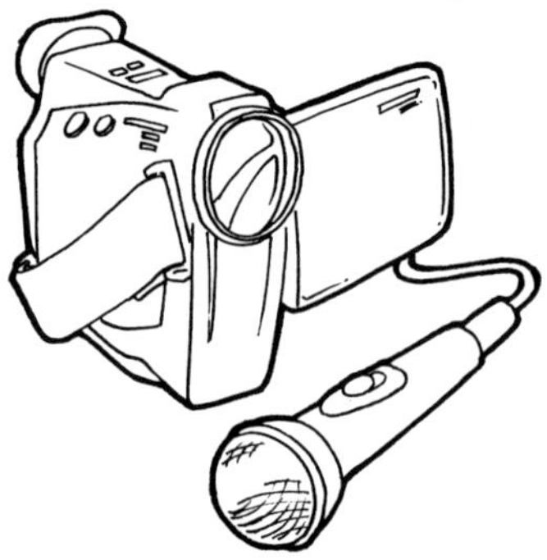

Registration of information (recording, microphone, video)

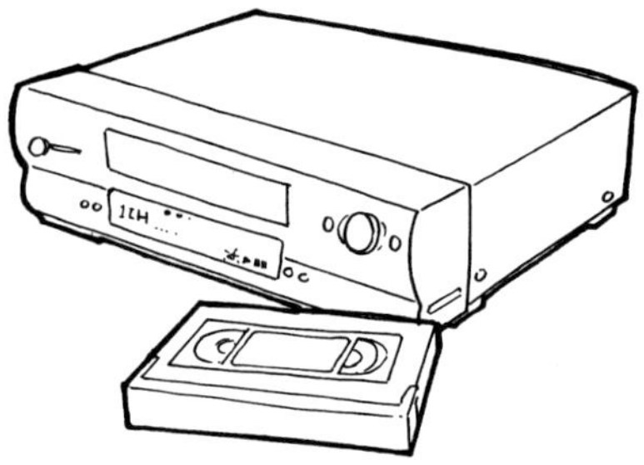

Temporary retention of information (cassette/video recorder)

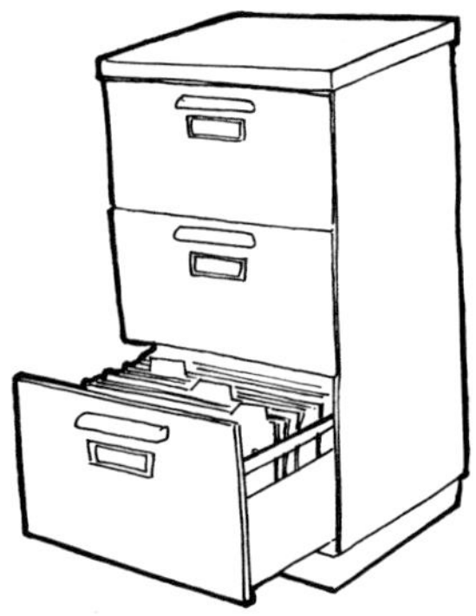

Permanent retention (long-term store, filing cabinet)

Memory is not a ‘thing’, but a process involving a number of stages.

- **Attention.** Attention is the mechanism by which information enters the brain. If you do not attend to information, it will not be encoded or stored.
- **Encoding.** Encoding is the registration of information at the time of learning. The strength of this registration or coding depends on the depth of processing, or on the amount of meaning associated with the information. Emotional events, or things you are interested in, are usually more meaningful, and are therefore processed at a deeper level – they become attached to existing memory structures.
- **Storage.** Once the information is encoded, it is stored in the long-term memory.
- **Consolidation.** If the information is not rehearsed or practised, then it will probably be lost. The process of practising is called consolidation. For instance, if someone tells you their phone number, you need to use it several times before you begin to remember it.
- **Retrieval.** Retrieval involves accessing the information stored in the long-term memory. Retrieval can be improved when given cues, eg, the nurse’s name begins with ‘B’, or when you are trying to recall something in the same environment in which it was originally learned.

Understanding memory

There are different aspects to memory, with a variety of often confusing names. Put simply, memory can be divided into time period involved (immediate, short-term, long-term and future) and information to be remembered (verbal, spatial, motor skill).

- **Immediate, or working memory.** This is the initial stage of memory. Information is taken in initially through the senses (sight, hearing, taste and smell). This information goes into the memory, where it is held for a very brief time, usually a few seconds. It can be viewed as a 'scratchpad' upon which we temporarily store information prior to processing or discarding it.
- **Short-term, or recent memory.** This is information that is stored just long enough to be used. It may be a few minutes, or hours, or days. The hippocampus area in the middle of the brain is thought to be important for laying down more permanent memories.
- **Long-term, or remote memory.** This is memory for 'episodes', or things that have happened to you in the past. It is also called 'episodic memory', or 'autobiographical memory'.
- **Prospective memory.** This is the ability to remember things for the future, and involves a certain amount of planning. For example, 'Meet Marina at 3.00.' This type of memory is thought to be closely linked to the frontal lobe area of the brain, where organising and planning is based.
- **Verbal, semantic or auditory memory.** This is remembering events using words. Words and language tend to be located in the left temporal area of the brain, so this is the area that is activated when, for example, you remember a story.
- **Visual, or spatial memory.** This is remembering pictures or images. When you remember pictures and images, it tends to be the right temporal area of the brain that is activated.
- **Motor memory.** This is remembering a particular motor skill, such as riding a bicycle, thought to be associated with the cerebellum.
- **Procedural memory.** This is remembering a 'procedure', such as how to switch on a computer. This type of memory often seems to bypass conscious control.

1 What are the five processes involved in memory?
2 Describe two different types of memory, and say roughly where they are located in the brain.

How relevant did you find this sheet? Very ☐ Slightly ☐ Not very ☐

Using external aids for improving memory

We all use a variety of 'external memory strategies' to help us remember things, whether we have had a brain injury or not. We might make notes; keep a diary; use a calendar or filing system, or just get into a regular routine.

Some simple measures can be taken to organise yourself, in the home or work place, in order to minimise the effects of memory problems:

(a) Adapt your environment:

- Keep a notepad and pen by the telephone.
- Put up a noticeboard, white board or memo board in a prominent place.
- Label cupboards or doors.

(b) A place for everything, and everything in its place:

- Have a key ring by the door where you always hang your keys.
- Have a special place where you put your wallet and glasses.
- Have an 'in-tray' for bills and letters, and a filing system for bills and legal documents.
- Place items strategically. For example, always put your umbrella on the floor in front of you when you visit the doctor; put letters to post by the door.

(c) Getting into a routine:

- Routines and good habits can ease memory difficulties.
- Pay bills on time if possible, or set up standing orders.
- Carry out certain activities on certain days.
- Keep a daily timetable on the noticeboard you have set up, and use it!

(d) Improve wellbeing:

- Anxiety, stress and depression can make memory difficulties worse, so it is important to look for ways to reduce these psychological difficulties.
- Put effort into maintaining friendships and developing new friendships. Talk about your difficulties.
- Plan positive, enjoyable experiences – seek out relaxing, pleasurable activities.
- Stay physically active and fit. Carry out some exercise at least once a day, even if it is just going for a walk.
- Be assertive. Learn to 'say no' to excessive demands, or things that are not important.
- Manage your time. Take breaks. Learn to relax and look after yourself.

Using external aids for improving memory

(e) **External aids:**

- ➤ **Diary/*Filofax*® notebook.** Make sure it is portable and possibly keep a larger diary at home to record the events of the day.
- ➤ ***Post-It*® notes and stickers.** Stick a *Post-It*® sticker to your diary each day, and write a 'to do' list.
- ➤ **Wallchart/wipe-off board.** This makes it visual. Use it for reminders of events and messages, and to help plan.
- ➤ **Calendar.** A large wall calendar is useful for writing down important appointments and social occasions.
- ➤ **Watch.** Use a battery-operated watch that can bleep to give you a half-hourly prompt to check your daily planner.
- ➤ **Dictaphone.** Use this to keep verbal messages, especially if you do not like writing.
- ➤ **Telephone answering machines** can help to reduce the problem of phone messages being forgotten or lost.
- ➤ **Make lists.** Writing shopping lists before going to the shops or to do lists to help you organize your day.
- ➤ **Mobile phones.** Useful for storing information such as important telephone numbers, used as a diary, notebook, alarm and mini dictaphone.
- ➤ **Use a pill reminder for medication.** Establish a routine of filling the pill organiser before bed (if it is for daily use), or on Sundays (if it is for weekly use). Keep it somewhere obvious.
- ➤ **Keep a kitchen timer by the cooker.** Alarms are useful reminders to start or stop a certain activity.
- ➤ **List telephone numbers.** Keep a list of important telephone numbers by the phone.
- ➤ **Investigate electronic pagers**, such as the *Neuropager* system.
- ➤ **Personal computers** are very useful for storing information.
- ➤ **Notes/memos.** Write important things to remember on memos, and put them in prominent places. For example, 'Turn off cooker', or 'Remember keys'.
- ➤ **Write on the back of your hand.** Sometimes just a letter of the alphabet is enough of a trigger.

1 Think of any other external strategies that you find useful.
2 Discuss which three external strategies you find most useful.

How relevant did you find this sheet? Very ☐ Slightly ☐ Not very ☐

Using internal memory strategies

Internal strategies are things that you 'do inside your head' to try to remember things. For example, thinking about something in a particular way, or trying to visualise something as a picture. Be realistic, and accept that after a brain injury you will not be as good at using these strategies, because your brain may have less capacity and flexibility.

Attention. Pay attention; focus on what is being said, and try to reduce background distractions. You will attend better if you are not tired, feel good, and want to remember.

Small chunks. Organise information under key headings, in small amounts. Try to break down information into small, relevant, simple, 'bite-sized' chunks or categories, rather than long, rambling streams of information. Put no more than five or six 'bits' of information in each chunk.

Repeat and rehearse. Repeat information over and over, silently in your mind. This is useful when trying to learn someone's name, or a telephone number.

Aim for 'deep-level processing'. The more the new information can be attached to existing memories or mental structures, the deeper it will be processed. For example, if a mechanic tells you that you have a problem with the camshaft on your car, and you understand the workings of an engine and know what the camshaft is, you are more likely to remember. If you have no idea what happens under the bonnet, the word 'camshaft' has no meaning: it doesn't conjure up any image, or fire neural pathways in your brain, and so you are less likely to remember it.

Make links or associations – 'deep-level processing'. Make mental associations in your mind, by linking new ideas to existing structures or information. If you want to remember that Charles's birthday is on 27 December, imagine that two days after Christmas, the poor chap probably got lots of joint presents as a child. The more links or bits of information, thoughts, or pieces of knowledge you have about something – however silly or bizarre – the deeper the level of processing, and the better you will remember.

Make visual pictures. 'A picture is worth 1,000 words.' We remember pictures and images much more than words. Thinking of somebody's name in terms of a picture will help you remember it. Try to make the picture as vivid, bizarre and exaggerated as possible – put colour, humour and movement into the picture. Thinking of a picture activates the right hemisphere of the brain; just thinking of a word uses mainly your left brain.

Mind maps or spider diagrams. These are ways of arranging information on paper so that it is easier to remember, because the information is broken down into a picture or map. The mind map has a number of routes, with sections of

Using internal memory strategies

information in small chunks. You can colour the routes, or put pictures on the map to aid recall. When your mind is searching for that information, visualise the map, and search the different areas of the map. What is in the top right-hand corner? What is in the bottom left corner? This technique is particularly good for remembering printed information such as notes for exams.

Question – 5Ws and PQRST. If you are trying to remember something, such as a newspaper story, ask yourself the five 'W' questions: 'What?', 'Where?', 'When?', 'Who?', and 'Why?' Break down information into those separate categories. Use these questions like 'coat hooks' to hang information on. The 'PQRST' strategy is also useful for remembering a story. The letters of the alphabet stand for particular instructions: 'P' for preview – take an overview, what it is about; 'Q' for question – line up your, 'what', 'where', 'when', 'who' and 'why' questions; 'R' for read; 'S' for state, or answer your questions; 'T' for test yourself.

Stories or rhymes. Make up a story or rhyme that contains the information you want to remember. Mnemonics are useful, such as 'Richard Of York Gave Battle In Vain' for remembering the colours of the rainbow (first letter gives you the colours in order – Red, Orange, Yellow, Green, Blue, Indigo and Violet). Making the rhymes or stories silly or funny can make them easier to remember.

The rhyming peg method. The rhyming peg method is a good way of remembering lists, and is a stimulating mental exercise. You need to learn a list of 10 images, or pegs, which rhyme with the first 10 digits. One = bun, two = shoe, three = tree, four = door, five = dive, six = sticks, seven = heaven, eight = gate, nine = wine, ten = hen. Create a vivid, exaggerated image of each of these pegs, and place the item to be remembered in the image. For example, make the bun as big as a double bed. Then, when you need to remember something, place it in your image. For example, if you want to remember a news item, say last night in the European football, Manchester United beat Barcelona 3-1, imagine the Manchester team in red, all lying in the bun, with the score 3-1 branded on the top of the bun.

Errorless learning. If you have a severe brain injury, you can learn more efficiently if you get it right first time. If you make an approximation and get the wrong answer, you are likely to remember the wrong answer rather than the right answer!

Expanded rehearsal. Repeat the information in your mind immediately after you have taken it in; then again after a slight delay. Then increase the delay by a few hours, and later by a few days. 'Little and often' is the best way of learning, while progressively increasing the gaps between rehearsal. This is also the best way of studying for exams.

Using internal memory strategies

Retrace by using retrieval cues. This involves retracing a sequence of events or actions inside your mind, in order to remember something. Mentally retracing your steps is helpful if you are trying to remember where you have put something.

First letter cueing. This is good for recalling somebody's name. Go through the letters of the alphabet one by one, and when you reach the first letter of the person's name, it sometimes prompts recall.

1 Discuss which of these strategies you use, or could use.
2 Why is it that if a football fan listens to the football results on a Saturday afternoon he will remember many more results than a person with no interest in football?

How relevant did you find this sheet? Very ☐ Slightly ☐ Not very ☐

How to remember new information – study skills

Environment. Ensure that your work environment is pleasant and tidy. It is sensible to have a specifically allocated work area that is well-organised and free from distractions.

Take breaks. Limit your study to short periods with regular breaks. People tend to lose concentration quickly after 50–60 minutes.

Build in rewards and treats. Treat yourself at the end of each of these study periods – perhaps to a cup of tea and a biscuit. Or do something different for 5–10 minutes – such as taking some exercise, or doing some chores.

Be selective in your reading. Try not to take on too much in one go. Pick out relevant sections and take brief notes. Always ask yourself, 'What is this person trying to say?', rather than just ploughing on through pages of text. Try to use the PQRST or 5Ws techniques described on page 23.

Make a plan or a timetable for study. Pin up this timetable in your work area, so that you can check you are doing the right thing. Take each subject and study it in separate blocks of study time.

Make mind maps. Condense your notes from handwritten text to spider diagrams, or mind maps, on large pieces of paper. Use different coloured pens, and number points. Activate the pictorial, right side of your brain. You can then further condense these large colourful sheets to numbered key ideas on index cards.

Use expanded rehearsal. Test your new learning straight after reading, then again a short while later, then again a little later, and so on – gradually expanding the length of time from reading to rehearsal.

Classroom note-taking:

- ➤ Just identify the important points or ideas of the lecture and write those down, rather than writing down everything.
- ➤ If you do not understand, then ask questions, or ask for clarification.
- ➤ Keep your notes organised. Use colours, or draw boxes, to highlight important points in your notes.
- ➤ If note-taking is difficult due to problems with speed of processing, then take in a tape recorder or borrow somebody else's notes.

1 What can you do to improve your ability to study?
2 How long can you concentrate before your concentration starts to diminish?
3 What can you do to improve your note-taking in lectures?

How relevant did you find this sheet? Very ☐ Slightly ☐ Not very ☐

INFORMATION SHEET 5a

How to remember people's names

Repeat the name to yourself under your breath. Mentally spell out the name, or imagine what the name looks like. Rehearse and register it.

Write it down. If you want to learn an important name, write it down alongside any distinguishing characteristics (for example, 'Bill – the next door neighbour'). Then cover up the name, and just look at the characteristic and see if you can remember it.

Make a picture or association. Try linking the name to the name of friends or relatives, or famous people. Or think what the name suggests to you. Obvious examples include Mr Brown or Mr Short, but use your imagination and Mr Unwin could be pictured as an onion. Create a bizarre visual image of the name, and then include the person in the image. For example, Bill, who is your neighbour, could be transformed into a picture of a face above the garden fence clutching a fistfull of bills. Joan could be Joan of Arc, dressed in all her armour. The more links you make with the name, the deeper it is processed and the easier it is to remember.

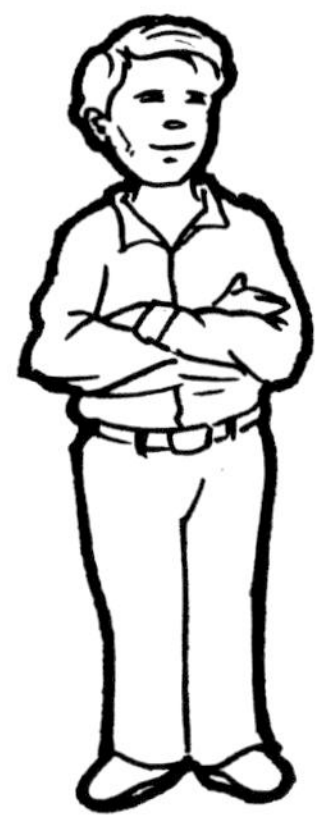

Mr Short

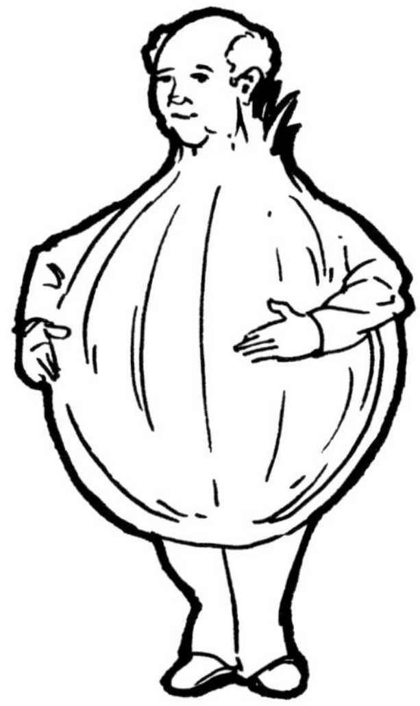

Mr Unwin

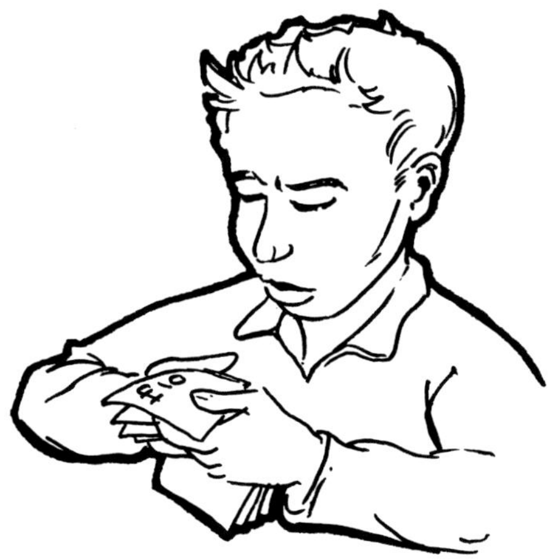

Bill

How to remember people's names

Pick out unusual facial features. Look carefully at the person's face, and sharpen your observational powers. Be aware of any prominent features, such as bushy eyebrows, long hair, or small lips. Whatever it is, form an exaggerated image of it, and then associate this image with the person's name. For example, you could imagine the person's bushy eyebrows as having hedges on their forehead. Then try to link the image to the name. Mr Norton's name could be remembered by imagining his eyebrows as handlebars of a motorbike.

Repeat the name back. Repeat the person's name back to them in conversation as many times as possible. This helps to imprint the person's name more firmly in your memory, and people like it.

First-letter cueing. If you can't remember the name, go through the letters of the alphabet slowly to try to prompt recall of the name. The letters act as a minimal prompt, and sometimes this is all that is required to aid recall.

Situational cueing. Try 'seeing' the person in a few different situations where you might have come across them – in the house, at work, in a shop. Imagining the situation can also prompt recall sometimes.

1. Think of someone you know, and make at least two associations with their name.
2. Describe what you can do to aid recall when you cannot remember someone's name.

How to remember to do things – prospective memory

Momentary intentions are spur-of-the-moment plans that you intend to carry out in the near or immediate future, such as going upstairs to fetch a hairbrush, or going to the toolbox to get a screwdriver. Strategies that can be useful for remembering momentary intentions are:

- Retracing mentally to the location where the intention was first thought of
- Using external memory aids – for example, a note, a list, or writing a cue on the back of your hand
- Positioning – place letters for posting by the door. When attending an appointment or meeting, put your bag in front of you, not on the back of the chair
- Ask yourself questions. What was I supposed to be doing? Who was it for? Why? When? Where?
- First-letter cueing – run through the alphabet and see if the idea pops up

Strategies that can be useful for remembering appointments or special events are:

- Using calendars, diaries and alarms
- Associating the appointment with what you will be doing immediately before and after it
- Making a visual picture
- Using mobile phones, or electronic organisers with alarms

Strategies for remembering chores and errands are:

- Using notes, calendars, memo boards and alarms
- Creating a story to remember the list of things to do
- Using the rhyming peg method to remember the list of things to do

1 John keeps losing his umbrella. What can he do to prevent this?
2 You have got to buy three items from the local shop. Identify three ways of remembering them.
3 Think of any other strategy that might help you to remember to do something.

How relevant did you find this sheet? Very ☐ Slightly ☐ Not very ☐

How to remember a route

Draw or purchase a map of the route you are trying to remember. Put landmarks on the map, and highlight with different colours. If you create your own map you will remember it better.

Write simple, step-by-step instructions for getting from one place to another. Use landmarks in the instructions. Practise following the route using these instructions.

Pick out and visualise memorable landmarks, eg, 'It is left after the red post box', or 'the car is parked next to the yellow ticket machine on the third floor'. Visualise and make associations for the number of the floor of the car park that the car is parked on.

Carry out the route with somebody else first, using your map, and then gradually do it on your own.

For finding your way in a building that you live in, place simple coloured tape markings or signs on strategic walls to indicate which route to follow.

Design and practise using a procedure in case of getting lost. For instance, a written cue card in the memory book, a telephone number, a mobile phone, or instructions to relay to a passer-by.

1 Identify three steps for remembering a route.
2 Identify three strategies for remembering where you have parked your car in a multi-storey car park.

How relevant did you find this sheet? Very ☐ Slightly ☐ Not very ☐

Learning to use a notebook or memory book

Portable with a pen. A small, portable book is best for people who are mobile.

Loose-leaf. It is best to use a loose-leaf diary or book, so you can insert or take out various sections according to your needs. The key is to start very simply, and build up gradually to a more complex system. *Filofax®*-style diaries are ideal.

Personalised book. When you have purchased a book, decide which pages and sections to include. It is best to remove irrelevant pages initially.

Emphasise the importance. If you can't see the need for the memory book, you won't use it. Identify five reasons why using the book is important, and write them in the front of the book.

Train to use the book. Initially this may just mean learning to carry it around wherever you go, as if it is part of your brain – the part that isn't now working. Once this habit has been established, practise finding each section in the book until you can do it quickly and easily. You will need plenty of practice in 'safe' situations that allow time for teaching, prompting and correction.

A typical memory book will contain the following sections:

- ➤ *Daily schedule* – to enable you to keep track of things you should be doing. It can also act as a record of what has been done.
- ➤ *Reference section* – this would usually include telephone numbers and addresses, injury information, and any other useful data that might be helpful.
- ➤ *Notes* – this usually consists of blank sheets: useful for notes or lists of things to do.

Look regularly. Many people find it useful to use an alarm as a cue to look at their memory book at regular intervals.

1 What is the best kind of memory book, and why?
2 Discuss the sections that you would like to have in a memory book, and how you would organise them.

How relevant did you find this sheet? Very ☐ Slightly ☐ Not very ☐

Notes for carers of people with memory deficits

Look after yourself. If you don't look after yourself, you will have less to give to the person with the problems.

Get into a regular routine. Develop and stick to regular routines for everyday activities. This helps to decrease confusion. People with memory deficits like structure to know what they are doing.

Provide an organised living environment. To ease the difficulties, ensure that the living environment is consistent and well organised. Have 'a place for everything and everything in its place'. Use external aids such as a calendar, memos and labels.

Provide an emotionally calm, relaxed environment. Try to ensure the living environment is calm, speak calmly, and try not to show your anxiety. Try not to take it personally, if the person forgets what you have said.

Break down tasks and information into small 'bite-sized' chunks. Present one piece of information at a time, rather than a lot of things at the same time. Avoid multitasking.

Memory is not an isolated problem. Bear in mind that memory problems do not often exist in isolation, and are often accompanied by problems of slowed thinking, executive skills difficulties, poor judgement, fatigue, lowered tolerance, and reduced emotional control.

Be patient. Give plenty of time to learn new things. Provide plenty of practice and repetition in a consistent way – you may get bored, but the person with the problem may not.

Remove distraction. Minimise distractions in the living environment, especially when imparting important information. For instance, switch off the television or radio when giving instructions.

Attention. Ensure that you get the person's attention when you are giving instructions or imparting important information. One way of doing this is to sit close to the person and maintain eye contact.

Keep it short and simple. Keep instructions short, and follow up with written information if necessary. Make sure you are clear what you are going to say before you start to speak.

Review and restate. Be prepared to review and restate information several times to help remembering.

1. Identify three things that would have an adverse effect on any individual's memory.
2. Make a list of the ways in which you could improve the organisation of the living environment.

How relevant did you find this sheet? Very ☐ Slightly ☐ Not very ☐

Memory quiz

1 How bad do you think your short-term memory is compared with before your injury?

The same ☐ Slightly worse ☐ Much worse ☐

2 Write down two external strategies that you could use to help compensate for your problem. For example: You have a doctor's appointment in three weeks time...... *Write on calendar.*

- ➤ You keep misplacing your keys in the house ...
- ➤ You forget what you went to the shops to buy ...
- ➤ You forget what you did last weekend ...

3 Write down two internal strategies or mental activities that you can deliberately carry out that may improve your memory for:

- ➤ Remembering somebody's name ...
- ➤ Remembering a telephone number ...
- ➤ Remembering a list of 10 bits of information for an examination ...

4 Explain why you are more likely to remember something if you make a visual image of it – for example, imagining Mr Baker made of white dough.

____

____

5 If you wanted to remember an article you read in the newspaper, what compensatory strategies could you try to use to remember it?

____

____

6 Give one reason why 10 bits of information laid out in a 'spider diagram' are more memorable than the same information written on a list.

____

____

7 What are some of the processes involved in memory?

____

____

How relevant did you find this sheet? Very ☐ Slightly ☐ Not very ☐

Remember a round

How difficult do you think you will find this exercise? Easy ☐ OK ☐ Quite difficult ☐ Very difficult ☐

Group instruction

This is a good exercise to start a group. Everybody has to give one piece of information about themselves, for the group members to remember at the end of the group. Use the lists below to give some ideas of the kinds of things they could say. The key skill in remembering each piece of information is being able to make a vivid visual image or association of the event with the person. The more bizarre and vivid the image, and the more it is linked to an aspect of the person, the easier it is to remember. Then see if you can remember in 30–40 minutes time. If you are not in a group, simply answer the following questions, and see if you can remember how you answered the questions some time later.

		Favourite	**Least Favourite**
1	Food		
2	Drink		
3	Television programme		
4	Film		
5	Book		
6	Singer		
7	Piece of music		
8	Holiday		
9	Job		
10	Politician		
11	Place		
12	Sporting hero		
13	Sport		
14	Animal		
15	Journey		
16	Hobby		
17	Personal achievement		

1	Where were you born?	
2	What is your biggest regret?	
3	What animal would you like to come back as in another life?	
4	What particular moment stands out in your life when you conquered fear?	
5	What would you do if you won the lottery?	
6	What have you always wanted to do, but been afraid to attempt?	
7	What luxury item would you take on your desert island?	
8	What one thing that others do irritates you most?	
9	What is your most embarrassing moment?	

Identify a positive event from the last week, and a negative event	
Positive	Negative

How did you find this exercise? Easy ☐ OK ☐ Quite difficult ☐ Very difficult ☐

Remembering sequences

How difficult do you think you will find this exercise? Easy ☐ OK ☐ Quite difficult ☐ Very difficult ☐

Group Instruction

These exercises are an ideal 'round' for starting a group, or can be carried out individually. They all involve remembering a sequence.

Alphabetical Shopping List. Make an imaginary-shopping list, with an item for each letter of the alphabet. Start with A and then B, and so on down the alphabet. Example: (a) Avocado, (b) Bananas, (c) Coke etc. In a group, each person in turn volunteers an item and everybody has to remember the whole sequence by the time you get to the end of the group. Then see if you can remember the sequence 30 minutes later.

Remembering an action or sound sequence. The first person performs a simple action or sound, which the rest of the group copies in turn or all together. Having gone all the way round, the second person adds to the original sound or movement which the group then copies. The game continues with the sequence getting longer and longer until all members have had a chance to add their own sound or action.

Remembering a verbal sequence in the form of a story. This is a variation of the above exercise, where one person starts off a story and each successive person in the group adds something to the story expanding the sequence. For example:

- That wine was delicious
- That wine was delicious Chardonnay
- That wine was delicious Chardonnay from California
- That wine was delicious Chardonnay from California. I also enjoyed the cheese.
- Etc.

Aunt Sally bought ... Remembering a verbal sequence in the form of a shopping list. (My Aunt Sally went to the shop and bought....) This is a good game to play on long car journeys. One person starts off by saying for example: 'My Aunt Sally went to the shop and bought a pint of milk.' The next person adds a further item: 'My Aunt Sally went to the shop and bought a pint of milk and a loaf of wholemeal bread.' Keep going for as long as possible. If somebody cannot remember the sequence they either drop out or the others in the group give them a prompt.

What strategies did you use for remembering those sequences?

How did you find this exercise? Easy ☐ OK ☐ Quite difficult ☐ Very difficult ☐

Remember a picture 1

How difficult do you think you will find this exercise? Easy ☐ OK ☐ Quite difficult ☐ Very difficult ☐

Instruction

Study the picture below, for one minute. Next, cover it up and try to remember what was on the picture. Use strategies such as chunking (breaking the picture into areas), linking, making associations, creating a story, visualising, asking questions, and rehearsing, to remember all the details. Then try to recall as much as possible immediately and 30 minutes later.

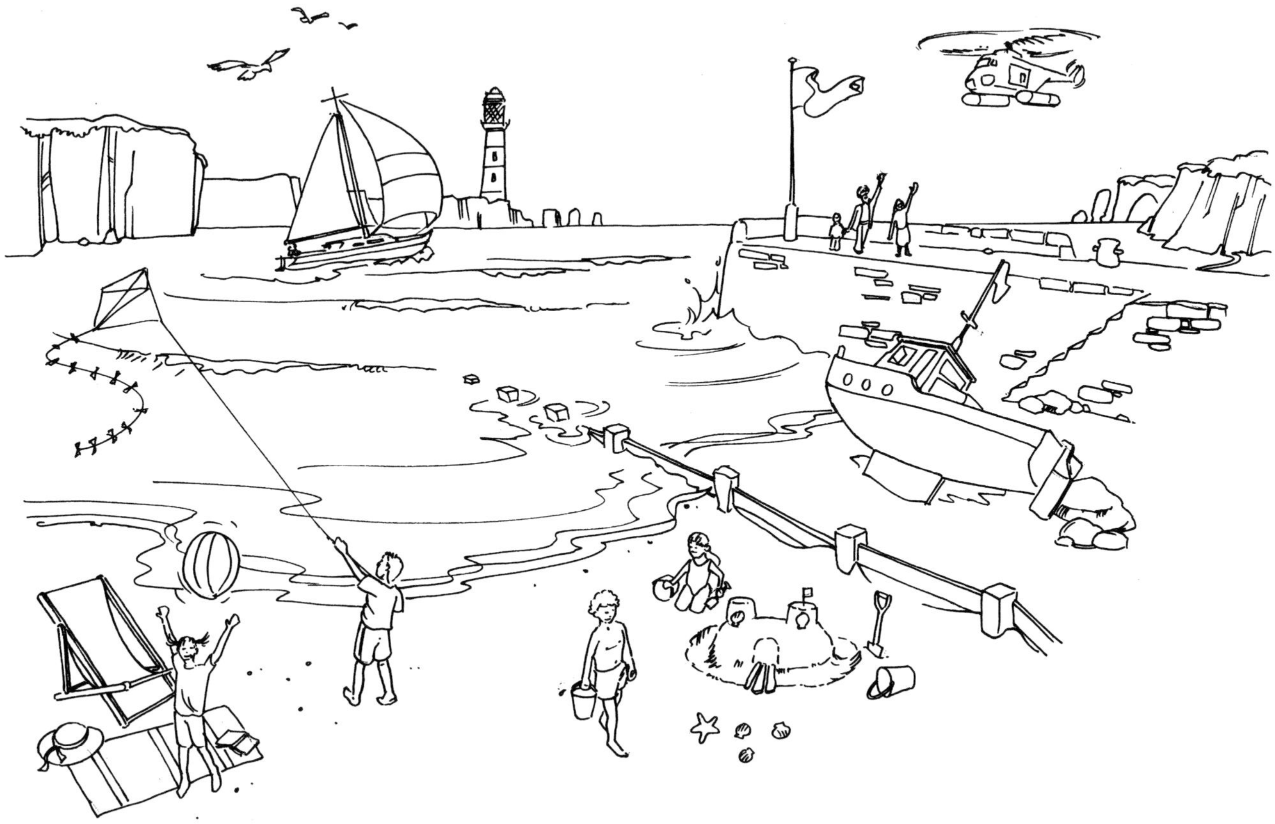

What strategies did you use to complete this exercise?

How did you find this exercise? Easy ☐ OK ☐ Quite difficult ☐ Very difficult ☐

Remember a picture 2

How difficult do you think you will find this exercise? Easy ☐ OK ☐ Quite difficult ☐ Very difficult ☐

Instruction

Study the picture below, for one minute. Next, cover it up and try to remember what was on the picture. Use strategies such as chunking (breaking the picture into areas), making associations, creating a story, visualising, asking questions, and rehearsing, to remember all the details. Then try to recall as much as possible immediately and 30 minutes later.

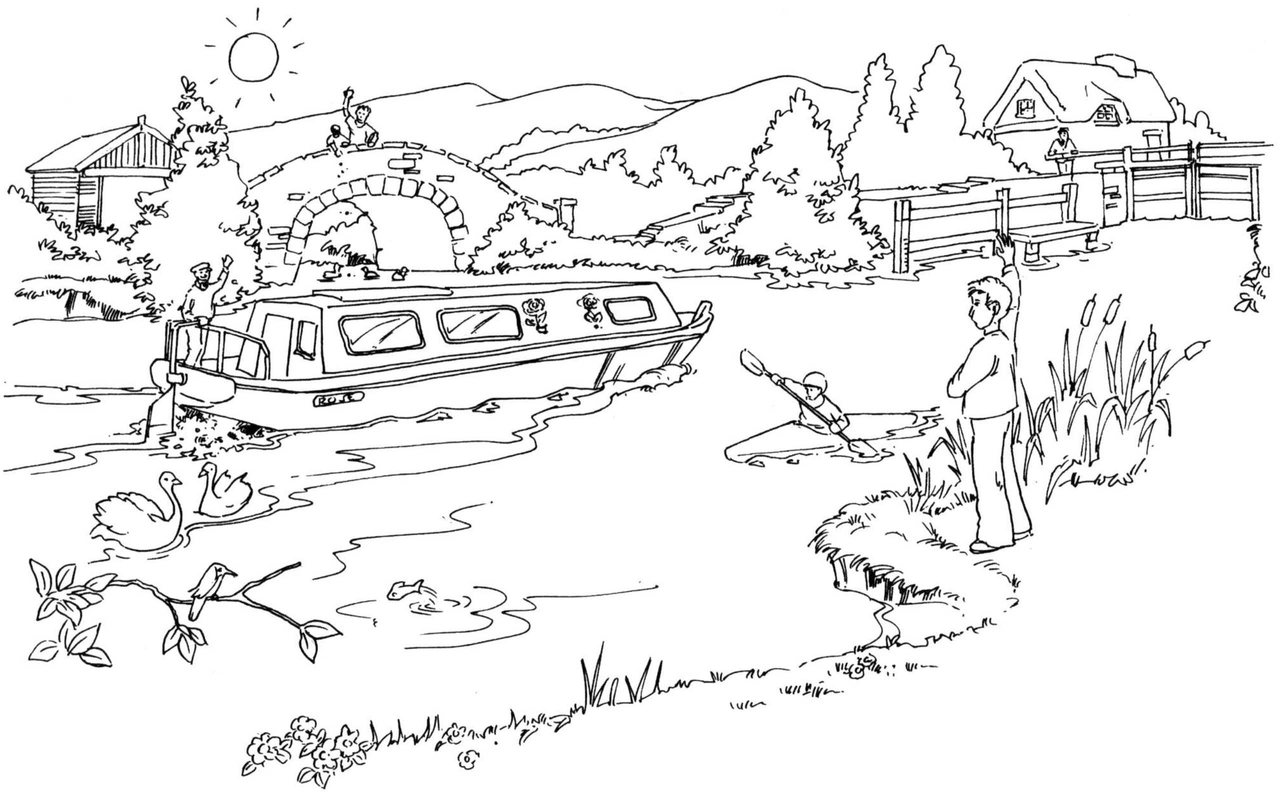

What strategies did you use to complete this exercise?

How did you find this exercise? Easy ☐ OK ☐ Quite difficult ☐ Very difficult ☐

EXERCISE 5a

Remember a name for a face 1

How difficult do you think you will find this exercise? Easy ☐ OK ☐ Quite difficult ☐ Very difficult ☐

Instruction

Study the names and faces for a few minutes, and then turn to the next page where the faces are printed without the names and see if you can remember the names. A few good strategies would include the following:

1 Say the name to yourself and make sure you have a clear mental image of the name.

2 Does the name suggest an image or an association to you? Make as many associations as possible.

3 Try to link the name to the face – pick out individual features – the more bizarre the association the better.

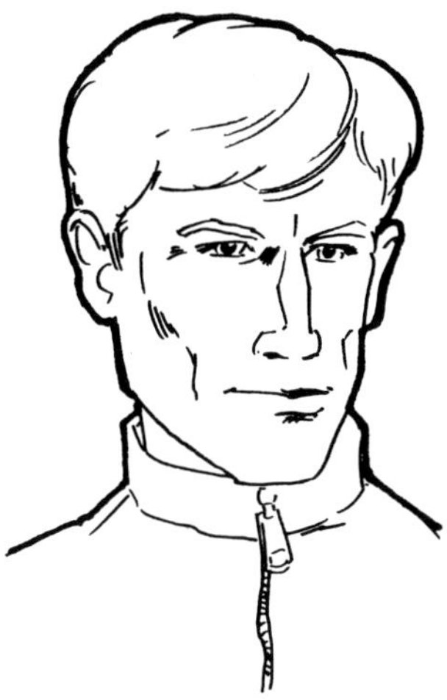

Tony Traynor

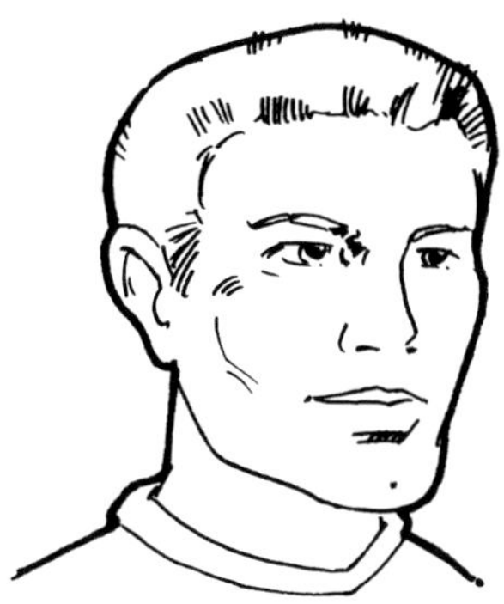

Jim Crew

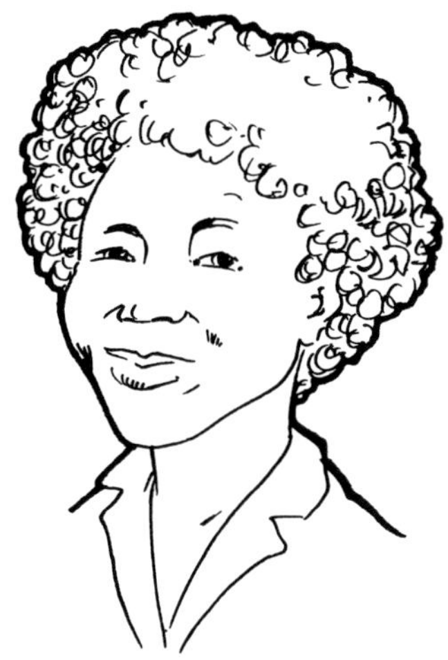

Miss Shirley Smith

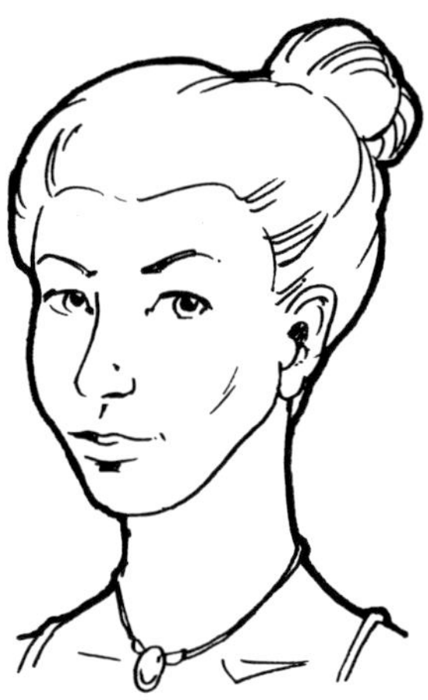

Mrs Ann Swann

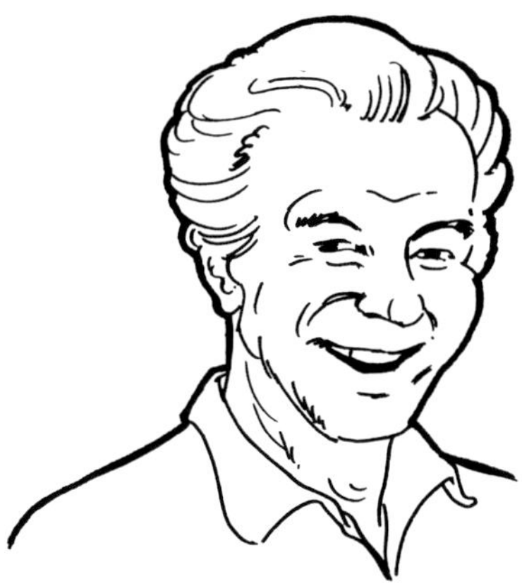

Mr Sidney Banks

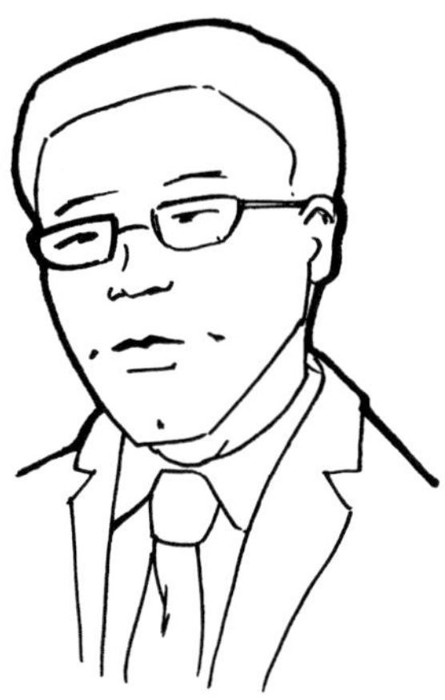

Mr Ono

EXERCISE 5b

Remember a name for a face 1

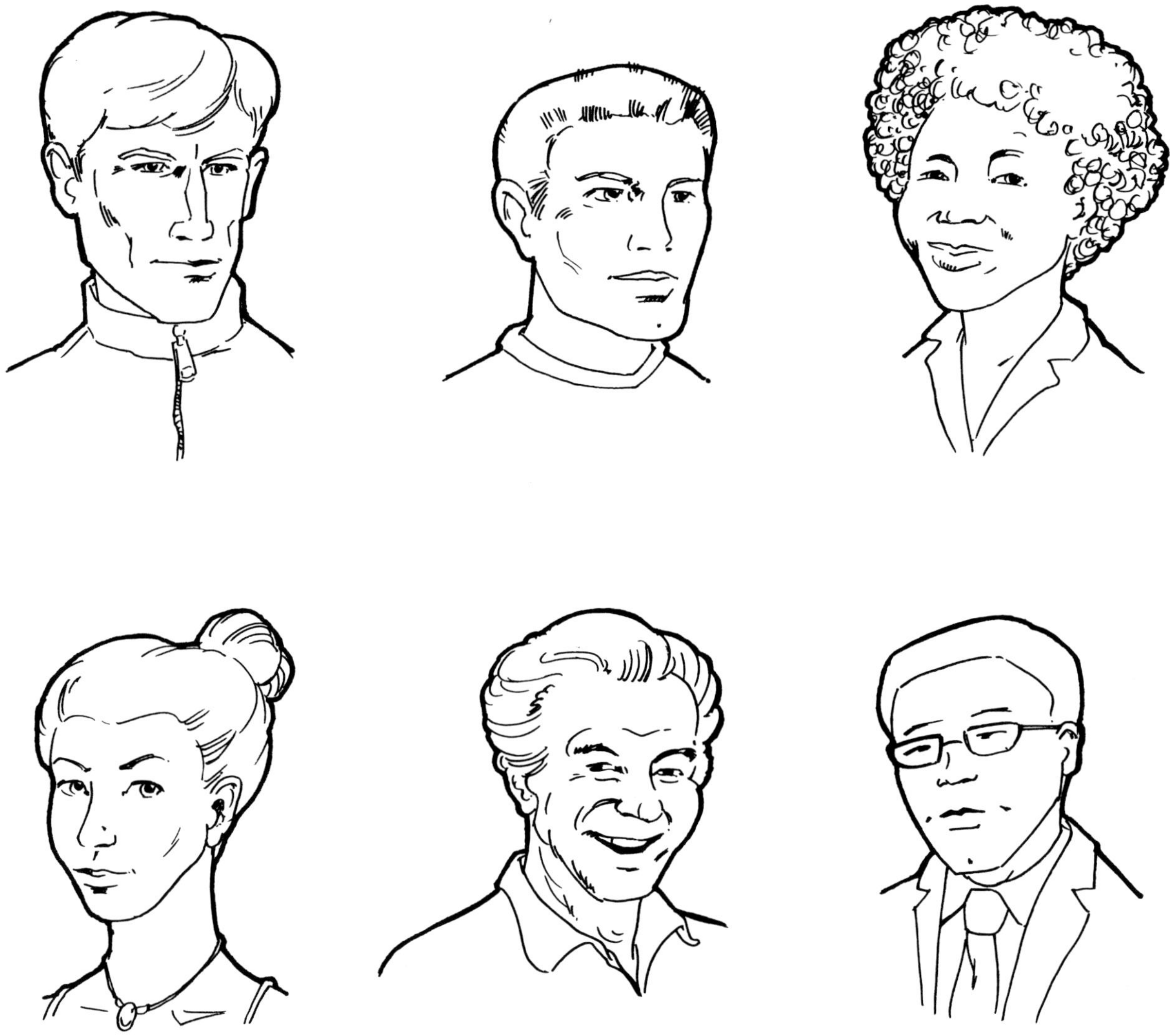

What strategies did you use to complete this exercise?

How did you find this exercise? Easy ☐ OK ☐ Quite difficult ☐ Very difficult ☐

Remember a name for a face 2

How difficult do you think you will find this exercise? Easy ☐ OK ☐ Quite difficult ☐ Very difficult ☐

Instruction

Study the names and faces for a few minutes, and then turn to the next page where the faces are printed without the names and see if you can remember the names. A few good strategies would include the following:

1. Say the name to yourself and make sure you have a clear mental image of the name.
2. Does the name suggest an image or an association to you? Make as many associations as possible.
3. Try to link the name to the face – pick out individual features – the more bizarre the association the better.

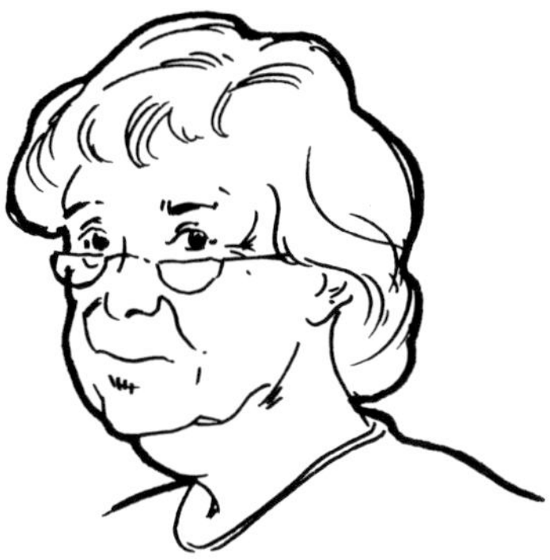

Mrs Iris Collier

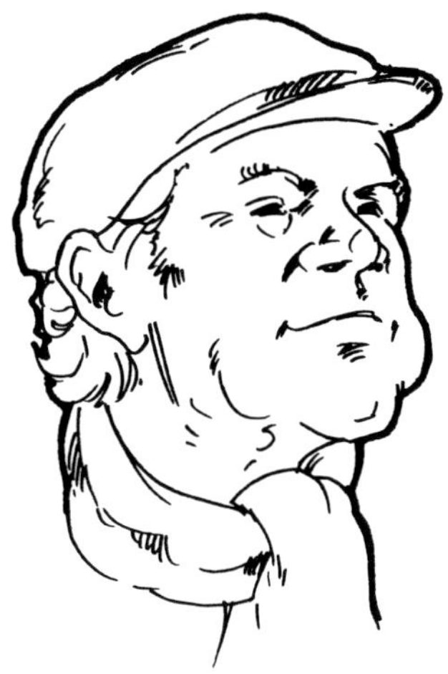

Jim Stevens

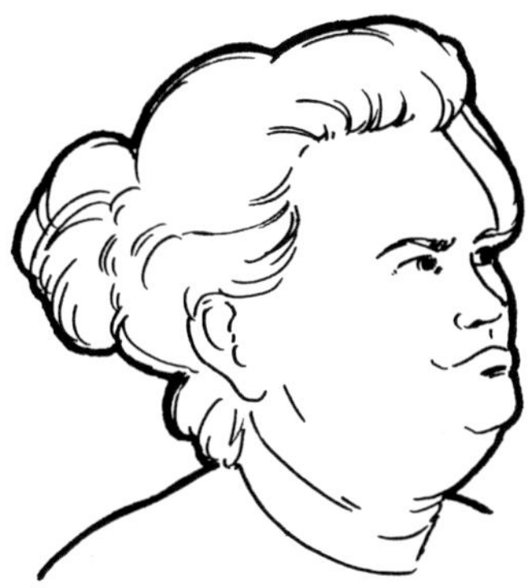

Rachel Ward

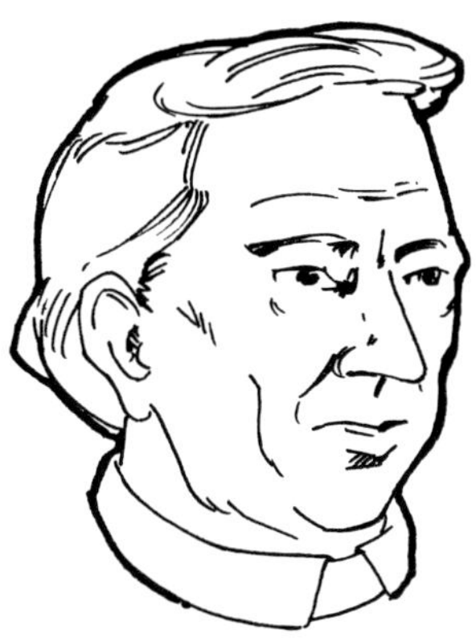

Mr Michael Hughes

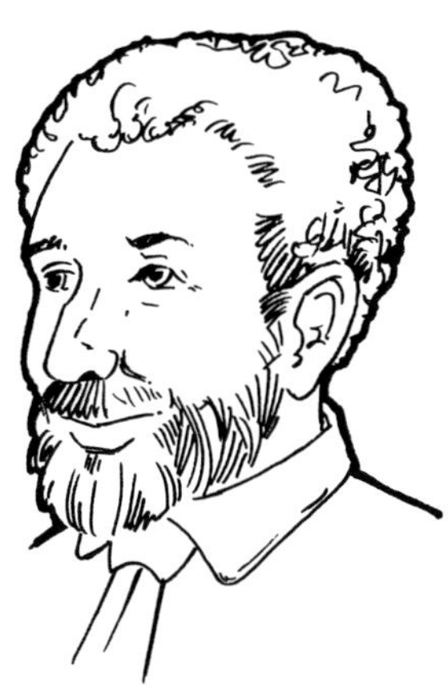

Dr William Foster

Remember a name for a face 2

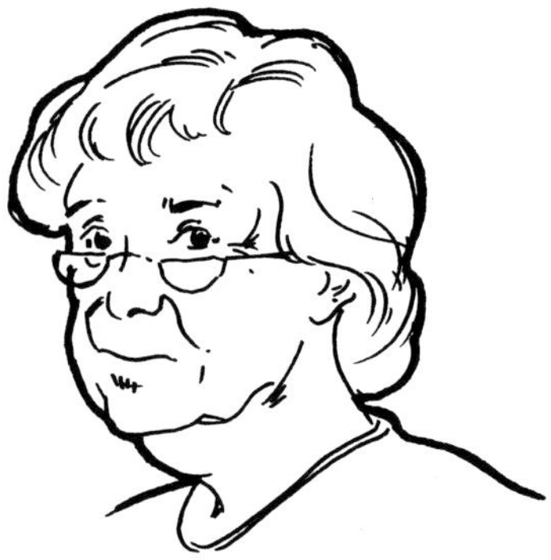

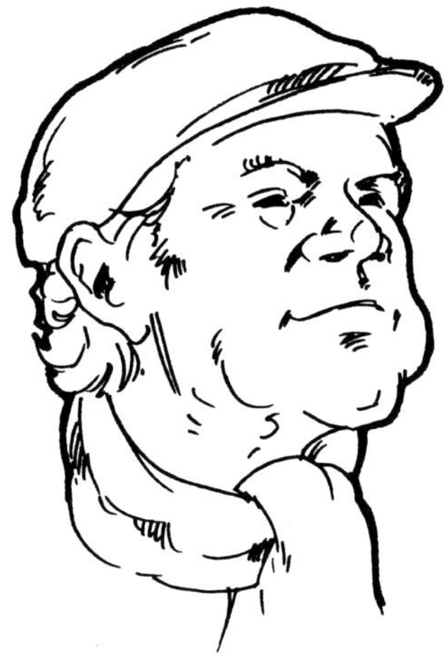

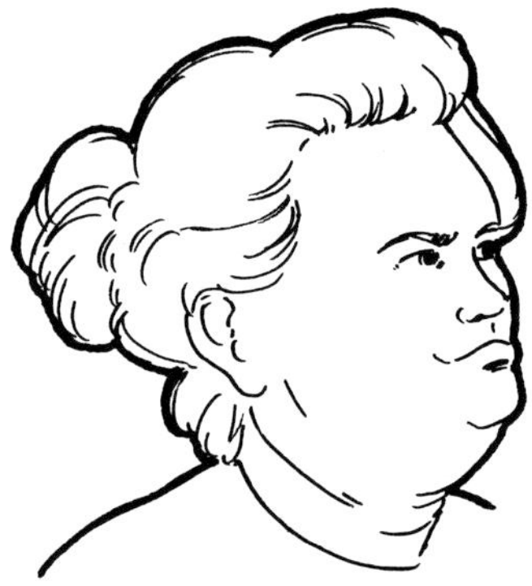

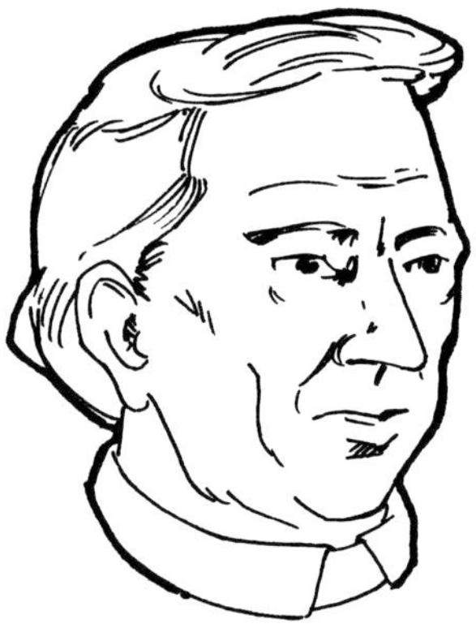

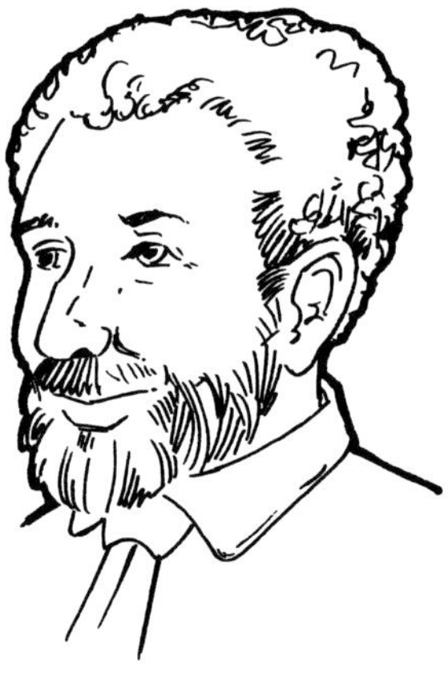

What strategies did you use to complete this exercise?

How did you find this exercise? Easy ☐ OK ☐ Quite difficult ☐ Very difficult ☐

Remember a name for a face 3

How difficult do you think you will find this exercise? Easy ☐ OK ☐ Quite difficult ☐ Very difficult ☐

Instruction

Study the names and faces for a few minutes, and then turn to the next page, where the faces are printed without the names and see if you can remember the names. A few good strategies would include the following:

1 Say the name to yourself and make sure you have a clear mental image of the name.

2 Does the name suggest an image or an association to you? Make as many associations as possible.

3 Try to link the name to the face – pick out individual features – the more bizarre the association the better.

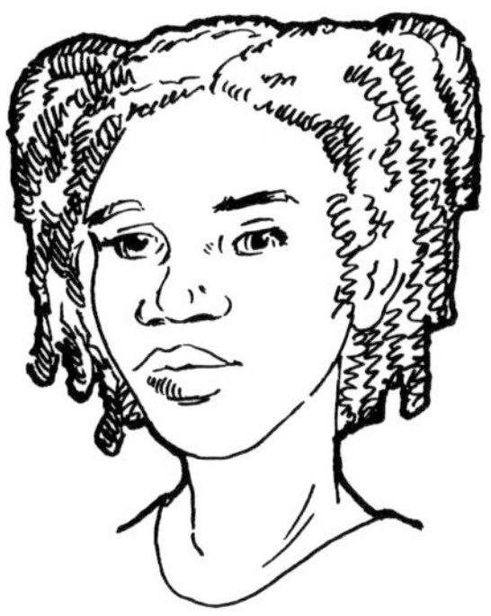

Sally

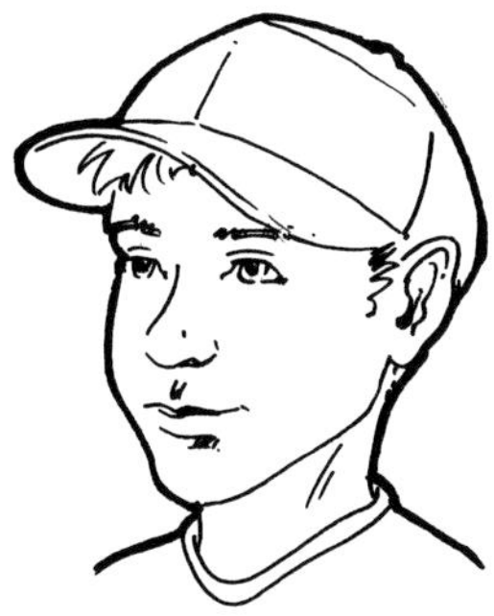

Ian

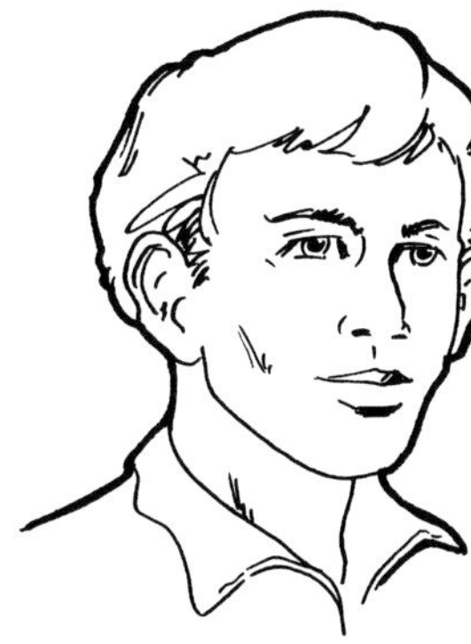

Charles

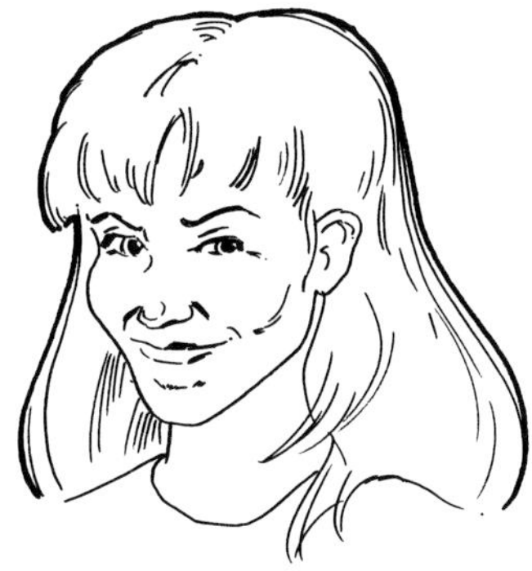

Jackie

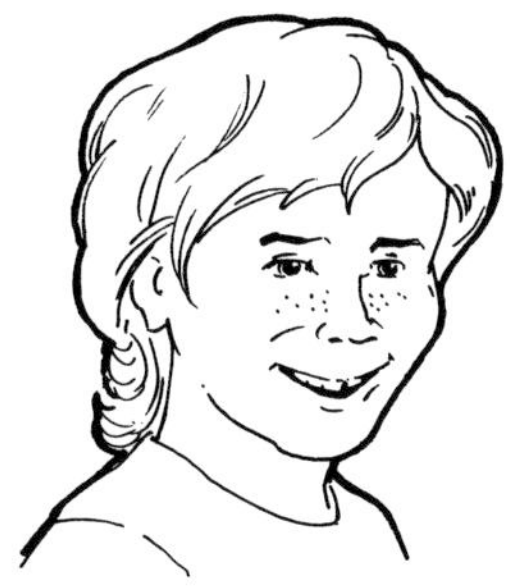

Francis

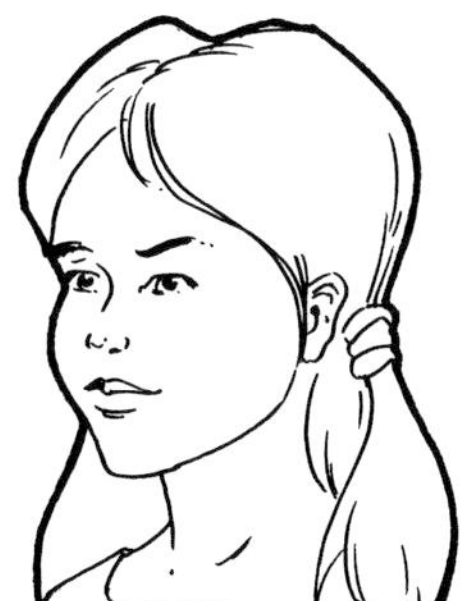

Carol

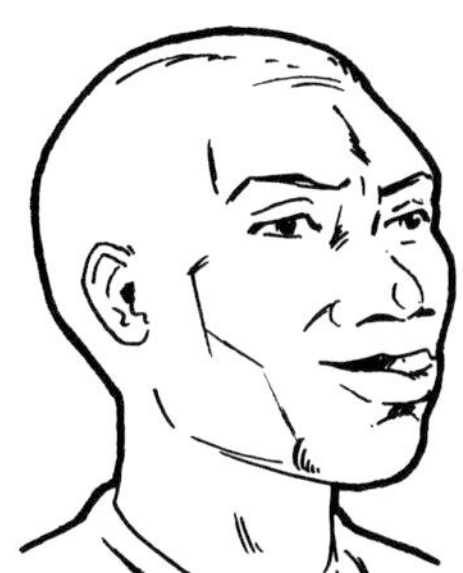

Jerry

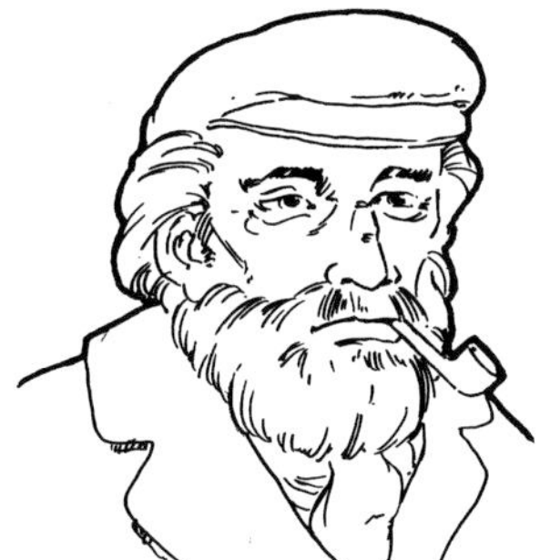

Alistair

EXERCISE 7b

Remember a name for a face 3

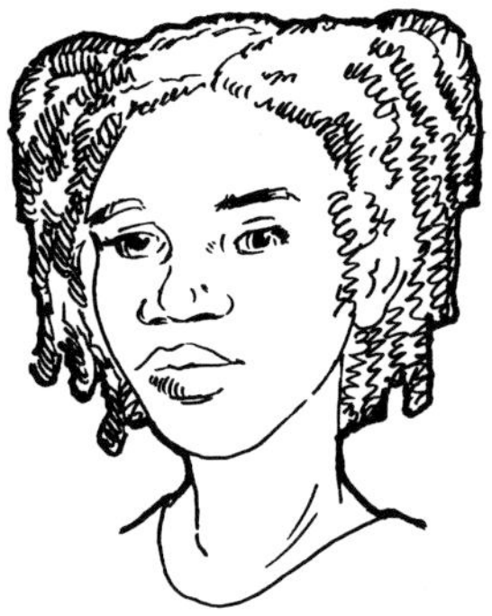
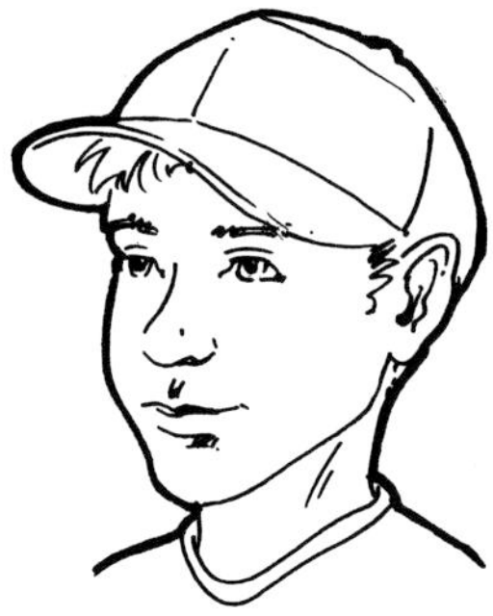
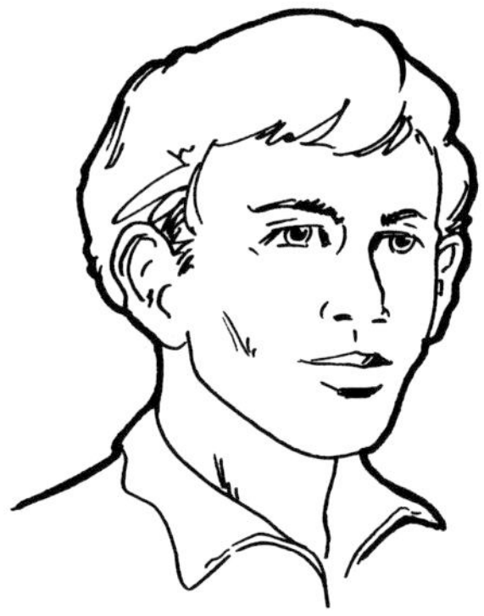
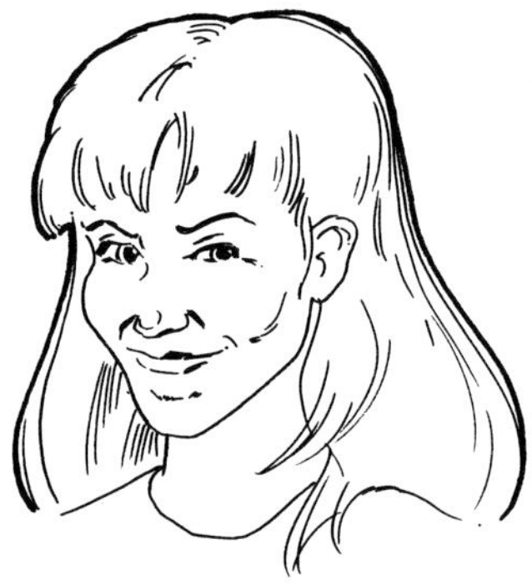
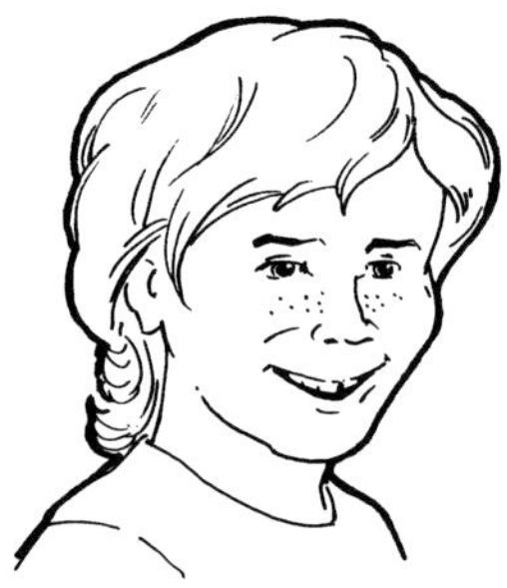
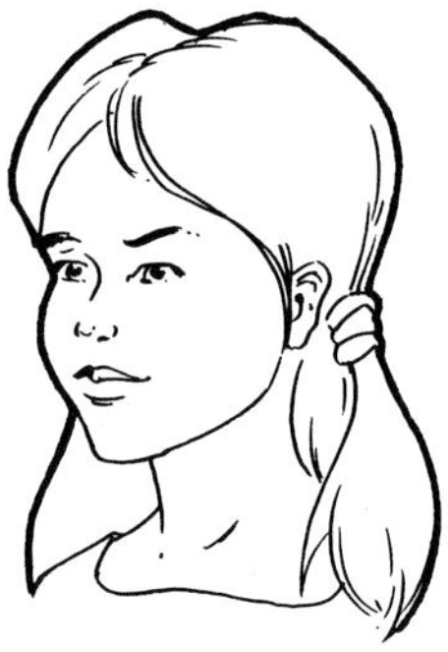
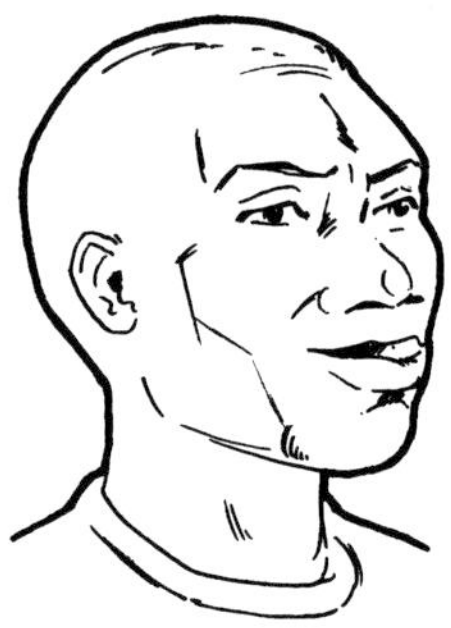
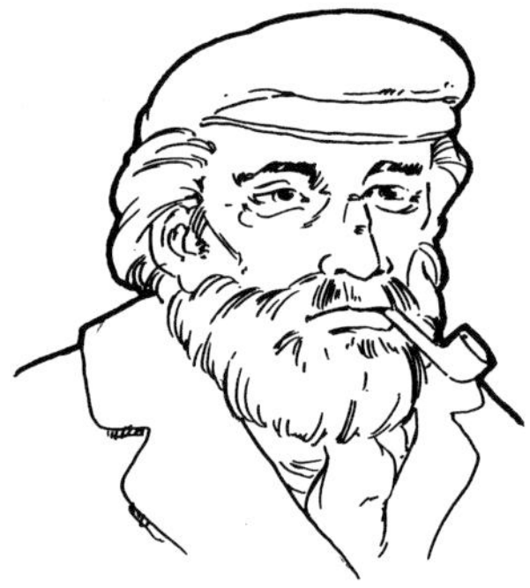

What strategies did you use to complete this exercise?

How did you find this exercise? Easy ☐ OK ☐ Quite difficult ☐ Very difficult ☐

Chunking – Kim's game 1

How difficult do you think you will find this exercise? Easy ☐ OK ☐ Quite difficult ☐ Very difficult ☐

Instruction

Try to remember these 12 items by breaking them down into chunks or different categories. There are four deliberate categories. Once you have sorted them into categories, try to link together the items in the categories with either a bizarre picture or a story. See if you can remember the pictures immediately, then 30 minutes later.

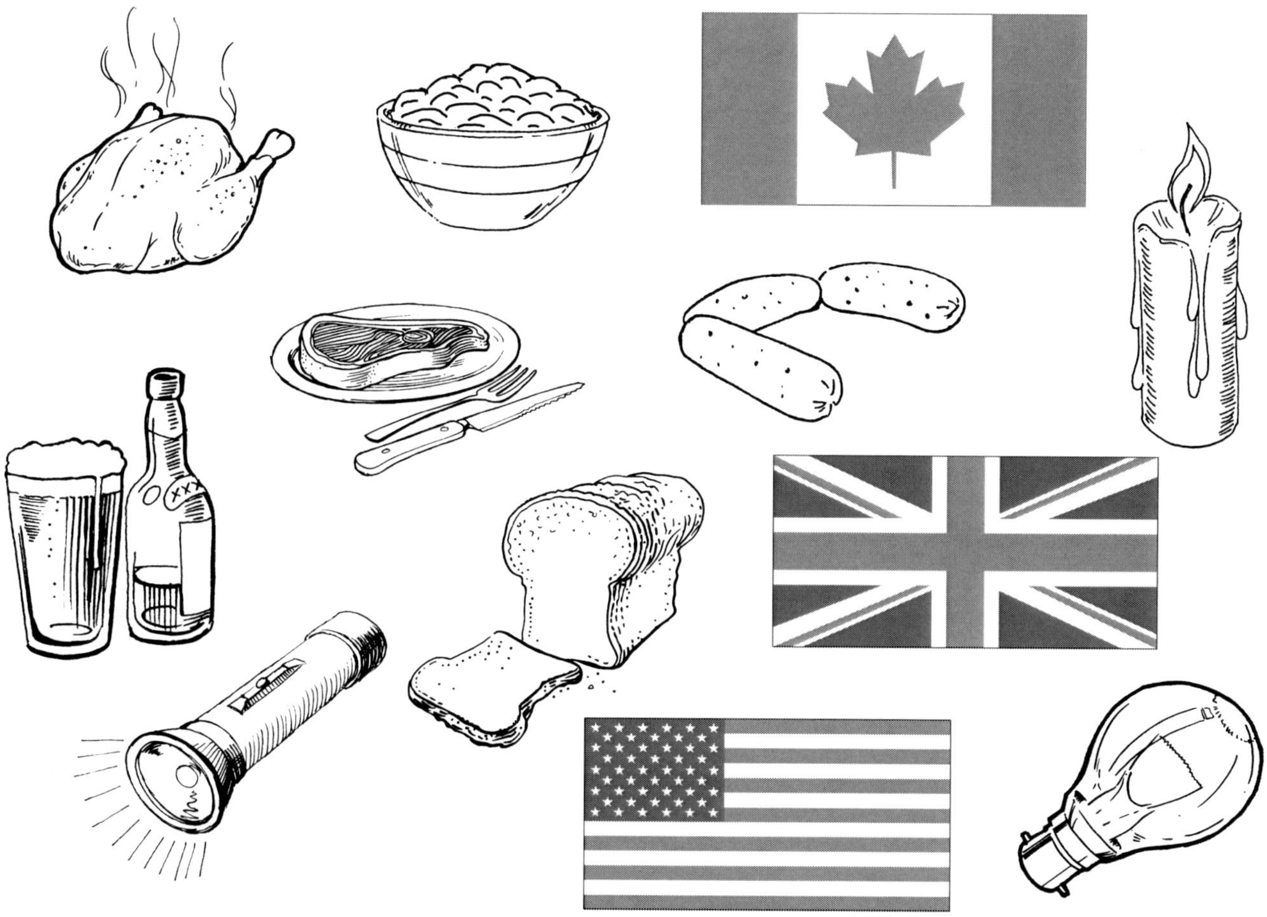

What strategies did you use to complete this exercise?

How did you find this exercise? Easy ☐ OK ☐ Quite difficult ☐ Very difficult ☐

EXERCISE 9

Chunking – Kim's game 2

How difficult do you think you will find this exercise? Easy ☐ OK ☐ Quite difficult ☐ Very difficult ☐

Instruction

Try to remember these 12 items by breaking them down into chunks or different categories. There are three deliberate categories. Once you have sorted them into categories, try to link together the items in the categories with either a bizarre picture or a story. See if you can remember the pictures immediately then 30 minutes later.

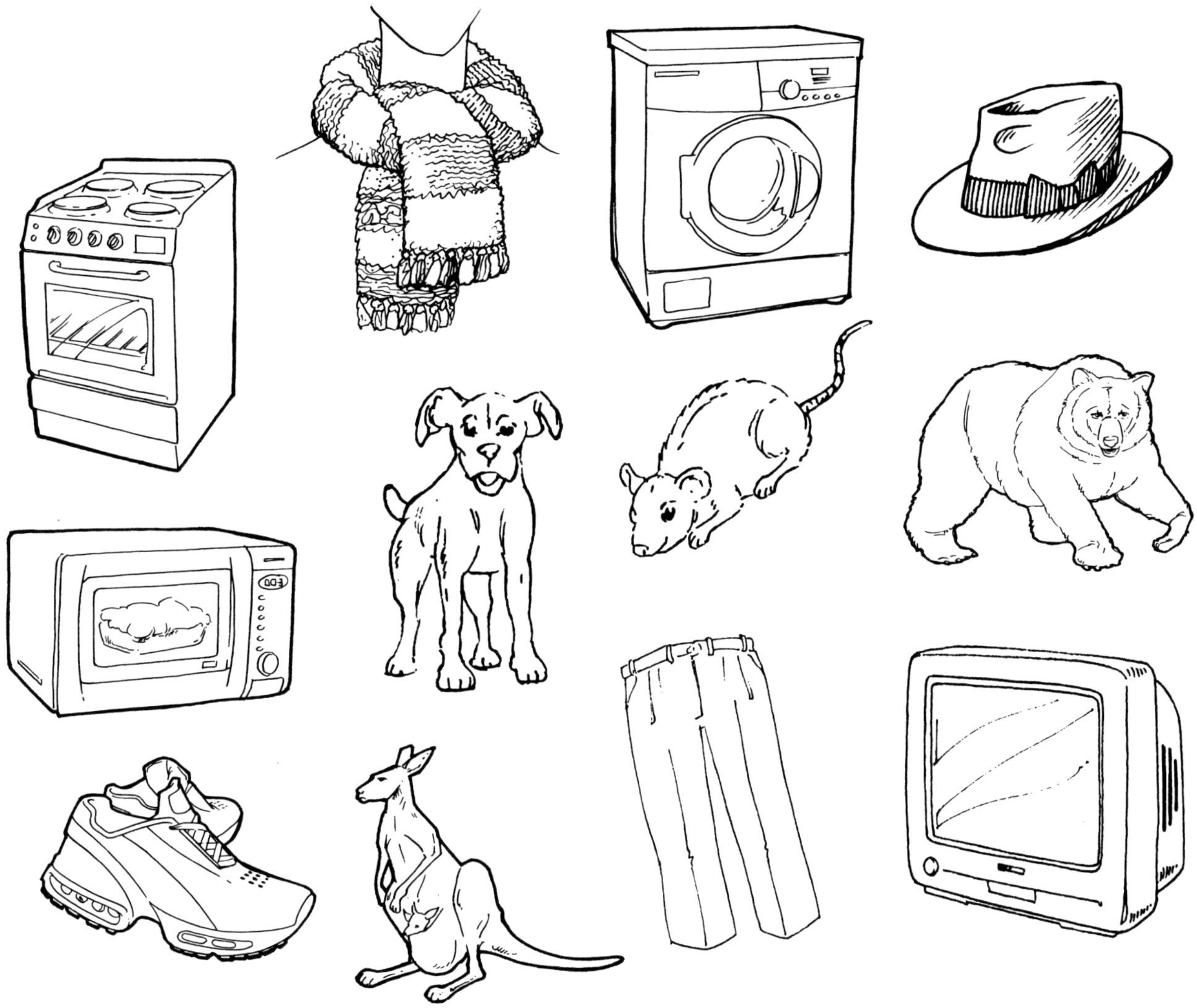

What strategies did you use to complete this exercise?

How did you find this exercise? Easy ☐ OK ☐ Quite difficult ☐ Very difficult ☐

Chunking – word list

How difficult do you think you will find this exercise? Easy ☐ OK ☐ Quite difficult ☐ Very difficult ☐

Instruction

Read through the following list of 15 words. How many do you think you will be able to remember? Now break up the list into three categories or 'chunks' (animals, jobs, clothes). Once you have sorted the items into their categories, try to link together the items in each chunk by making an association, creating a story, or creating a visual image.

List

Cat	Postman	Sock
Mouse	Lawyer	Trousers
Elephant	Hat	Secretary
Tie	Snake	Electrician
Wellington boots	Politician	Swan

What strategies did you use to complete this exercise?

How did you find this exercise? Easy ☐ OK ☐ Quite difficult ☐ Very difficult ☐

EXERCISE 11

News story 1: Driving down the wrong side of the motorway

How difficult do you think you will find this exercise? Easy ☐ OK ☐ Quite difficult ☐ Very difficult ☐

Instruction

Read the paragraph below, and then try to remember as much about it as possible. There are various strategies for helping: P = Preview – take a brief overview on what it's about. Q = Question – ask yourself key questions, such as 'Who?', 'Where?', 'Why?', 'When?', 'What?' Arrange these questions in the form of a spider diagram to make the answers more memorable. R = Read. S = State – state the answers to the questions. T = Test – just briefly test yourself that you have the answers to all the questions. Test yourself again in 20 minutes time.

Drunken Motorist Drives the Wrong Way

An electrician drove six miles the wrong way down the M4 motorway after downing pints of lager, a court heard. Harold Bishop, 34, had gone on a bender after splitting up with his wife two days before. Motorists had to swerve out of the way as he careered along blissfully unaware that he was on the wrong side of the road. Maidenhead court heard how Bishop, an electrician and father of three, had spent Wednesday night drinking with friends in The Boars Head pub before driving off in his Bedford van. He was stopped at Junction 11, shortly before 2am. Susan Bridges, prosecuting, said Bishop had been more than three times over the drink-drive limit. Magistrates adjourned the case until next month for pre-sentence reports.

Remember: P, Q, R, S, T.

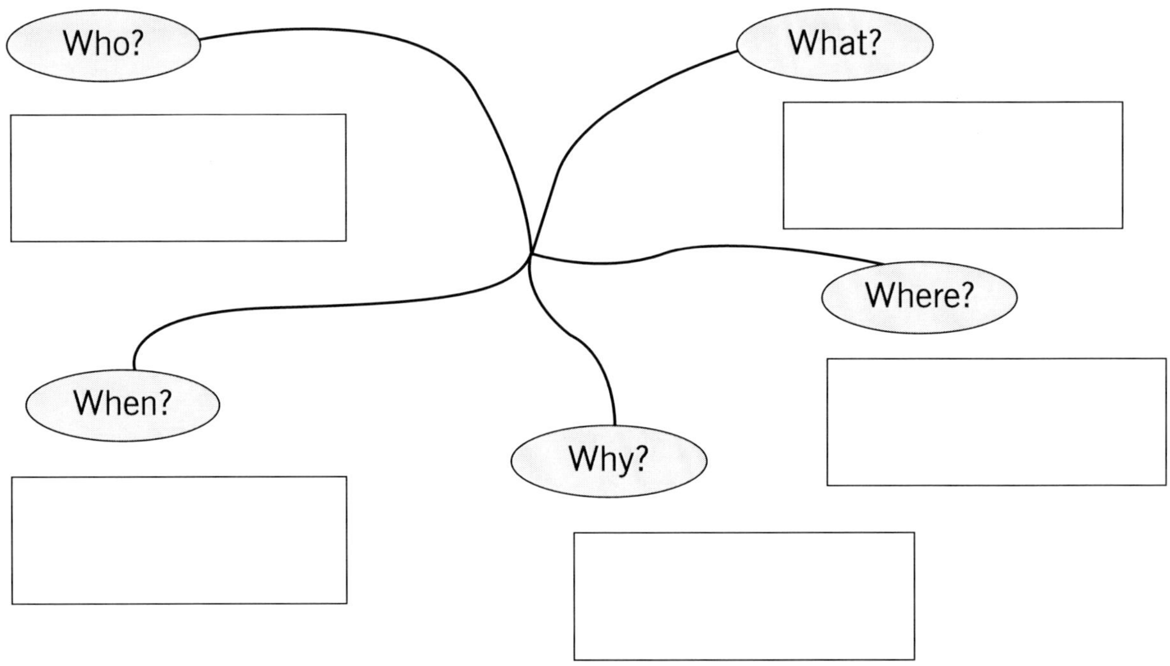

How did you find this exercise? Easy ☐ OK ☐ Quite difficult ☐ Very difficult ☐

EXERCISE 12

News story 2: Bees invade home

How difficult do you think you will find this exercise? Easy ☐ OK ☐ Quite difficult ☐ Very difficult ☐

Instruction

You have read an interesting story in the newspaper, and want to remember it to tell it to a friend. Try to remember as much as you can by using the spider diagram – write the key points in the box under the headings 'Who?', 'What?', 'Where?', 'When?' and 'Why?' If you break it down into these chunks you will have a better chance of remembering it.

Nightmare Weekend as Bees Invade Home

Neighbours were the first to spot the swarm over the chimney of Frank and Mandy Clark's home in Reading. Before they could alert the family the invaders had entered the kitchen and spare bedroom – and the Clarks had 6,000 honeybees as weekend guests. Mandy said, 'It was like a horror movie, they were crawling out between the skirting board and the carpet. The brickwork was completely covered in a moving black mass. They were buzzing so loudly we could not hear the television.' The council's emergency help line had little to offer, as it was the weekend and there was just a recorded message. On the Saturday night the couple eventually left the bees and went to stay at a friend's house. Bob Phillips – environmental health team leader for the council said: 'Pest control is not a statutory function of the council, and local people have the option of calling out private companies. The Clarks did the right thing, as if they had threatened the swarm in any way they might have attacked as one.' On the Monday morning an environmental health officer smoked out the invaders.

Remember: P, Q, R, S, T.

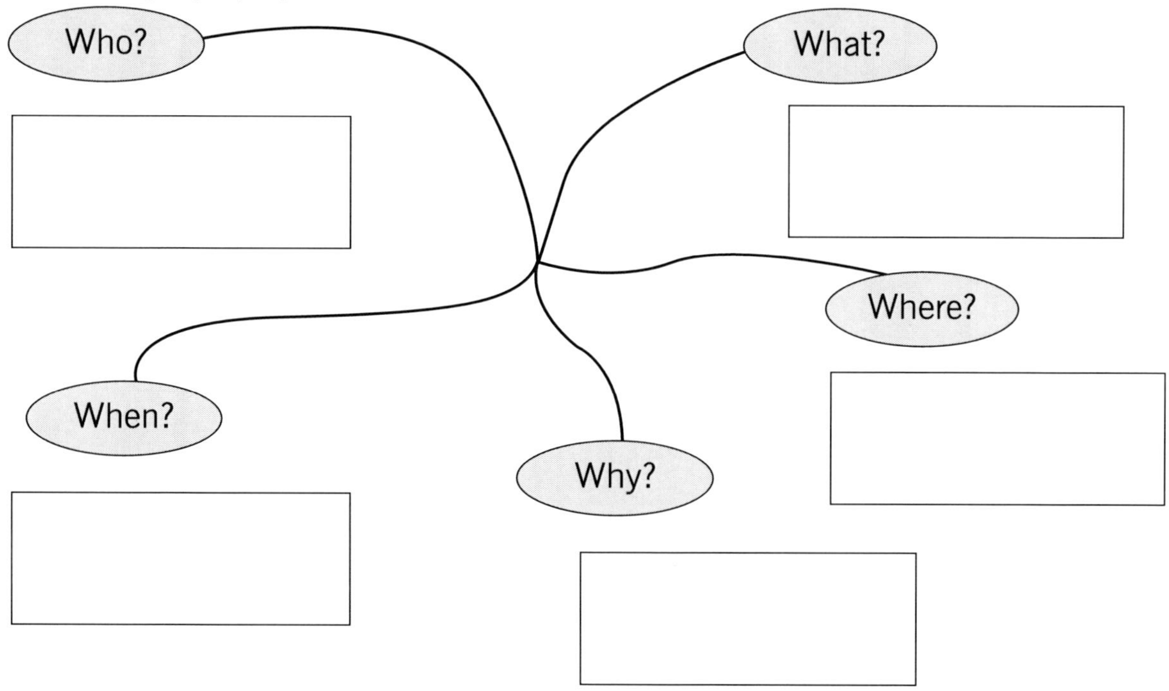

How did you find this exercise? Easy ☐ OK ☐ Quite difficult ☐ Very difficult ☐

Who is on the course?

How difficult do you think you will find this exercise? Easy ☐ OK ☐ Quite difficult ☐ Very difficult ☐

Instruction

Imagine that tomorrow you have to run a training course. You have been given a list of eight delegates, but you are worried that you will not be able to remember their names. First, organise their names on paper to make them more memorable, by using a spider diagram as shown. This will help you to create a more striking visual image than a list, help you to process the information more deeply, and create more cues for retrieval. When drawing your spider diagram, chunk information together into small groups, such as the four different employers who have sent the delegates on the course. Then try to visualise groupings and names, and try to make associations – eg, imagine a Carol Ward as a nurse on a ward, possibly singing a carol. Make your own spider diagram and work on ways to remember the names, then see what you remember 20 minutes later.

Computer training course – basic keyboard skills

Mr A Brown – *Evening Post* Newspaper
Mr C Davis – Reading District Council
Miss Jane Evans – Wokingham District Council
Dr Susan Flowers – NHS
Miss Jackie Hughes – Wokingham District Council
Mr D Marshall – Reading District Council
Mrs Sylvia Moore – *Evening Post* Newspaper
Mrs Carol Ward – NHS

Example of spider diagram

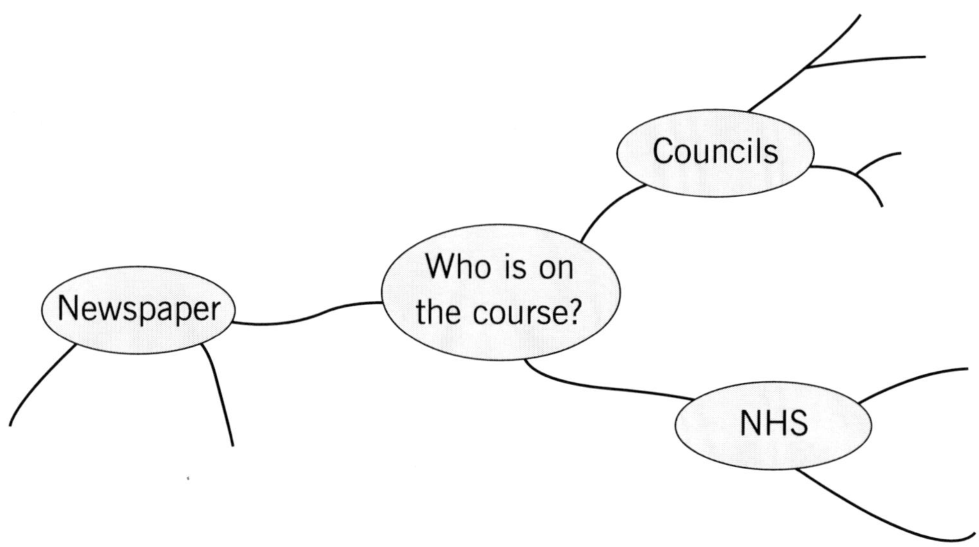

How did you find this exercise? Easy ☐ OK ☐ Quite difficult ☐ Very difficult ☐

Rhyming peg images

How difficult do you think you will find this exercise? Easy ☐ OK ☐ Quite difficult ☐ Very difficult ☐

Instruction

The rhyming peg method is a good way of remembering lists, and is itself a stimulating mental exercise. A list of 10 images, or pegs, which rhyme with the first 10 digits needs to be learnt. One = bun, two = shoe, three = tree, etc. Create a vivid, exaggerated image – for example, make the bun as big as a double bed. Then, when you need to remember something, place it in your image. For example, if you want to remember a news item – say last night in the European football Manchester United beat Barcelona 3-1 – imagine the Manchester team in red all lying in the bun, with the score 3-1 branded on the top. The more vivid and bizarre you make your image the easier it will be to remember.

1 Draw up a list of 10 things that have happened in the news over the last few weeks, then try to remember them using this technique.
2 Draw up a list of 10 items to buy from the shop.
3 Give a talk consisting of 10 points, that you will try to remember using this technique.

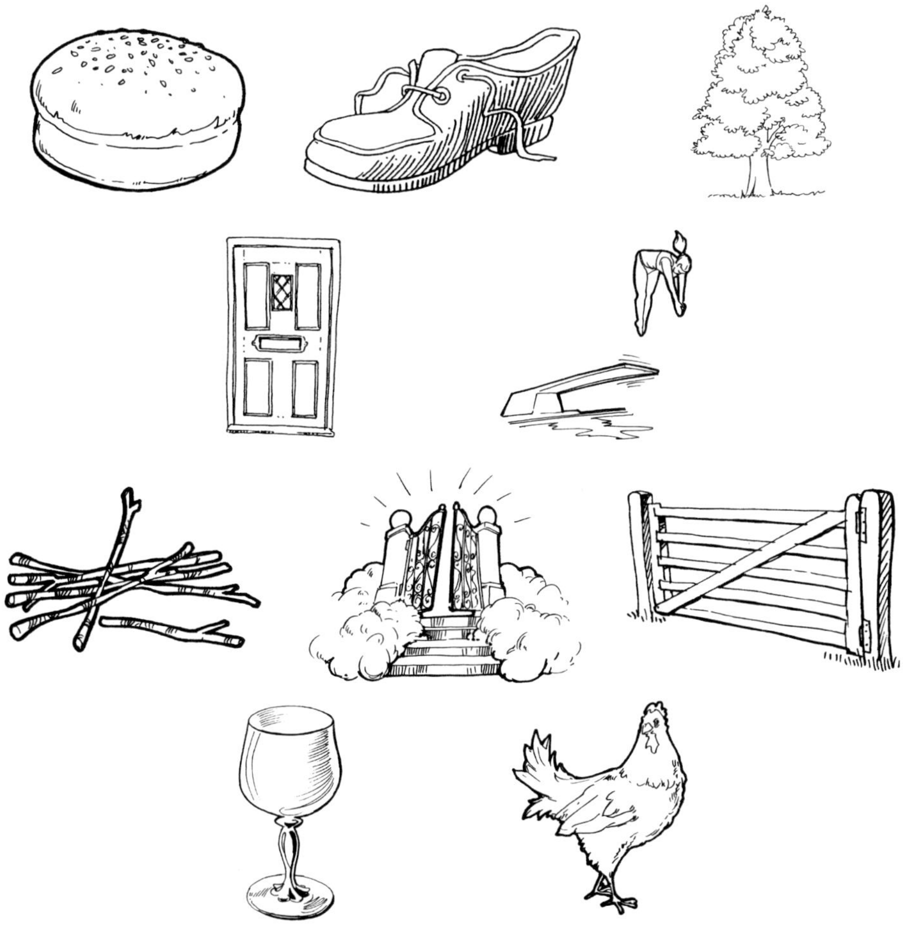

1 = Bun
2 = Shoe
3 = Tree
4 = Door
5 = Dive
6 = Sticks
7 = Heaven
8 = Gate
9 = Wine
10 = Hen

How did you find this exercise? Easy ☐ OK ☐ Quite difficult ☐ Very difficult ☐

EXERCISE 15

Visualise your house

How difficult do you think you will find this exercise? Easy ☐ OK ☐ Quite difficult ☐ Very difficult ☐

Instruction

Imagine the ground-floor plan of your house, and try to draw it like an architect's plan or map. Once you have drawn the map of your house, identify seven special places in your house, where you could mentally place things to remember them – mark these places on the map: eg, front door step, in the fridge. Imagine walking around the seven places in order – visualise them in your mind. Then imagine placing things that you need to remember in those special places. For example, the first item to remember is a large brown loaf of bread. Imagine a huge, exaggerated loaf sitting on the doorstep, that you have to climb over to get in. The second item might be a bunch of celery, so imagine giant sticks of celery lying on the foot of the stairs.

1 Draw a plan of the downstairs of your home.
2 Mark in seven places that you will use as 'pegs' to remember items.

3 Try to remember the following list by placing each item in a special place. Create bizarre exaggerated visual images. List: (1) A brown loaf of bread, (2) Celery, (3) 6 tomatoes, (4) A newspaper, (5) 12 eggs, (6) a tin of rice pudding, (7) A jar of strawberry jam.
4 Now try to do the same thing with seven items from the recent news.

How did you find this exercise? Easy ☐ OK ☐ Quite difficult ☐ Very difficult ☐

EXERCISE 16

Linking visual images

How difficult do you think you will find this exercise? Easy ☐ OK ☐ Quite difficult ☐ Very difficult ☐

Instruction

Study the sets of pictures below, then cover them up or remove them and try to remember what the pictures were. Use the techniques of making associations, or linking each picture together in a story as a way of remembering. The more bizarre and ridiculous the story, the better you will remember it.

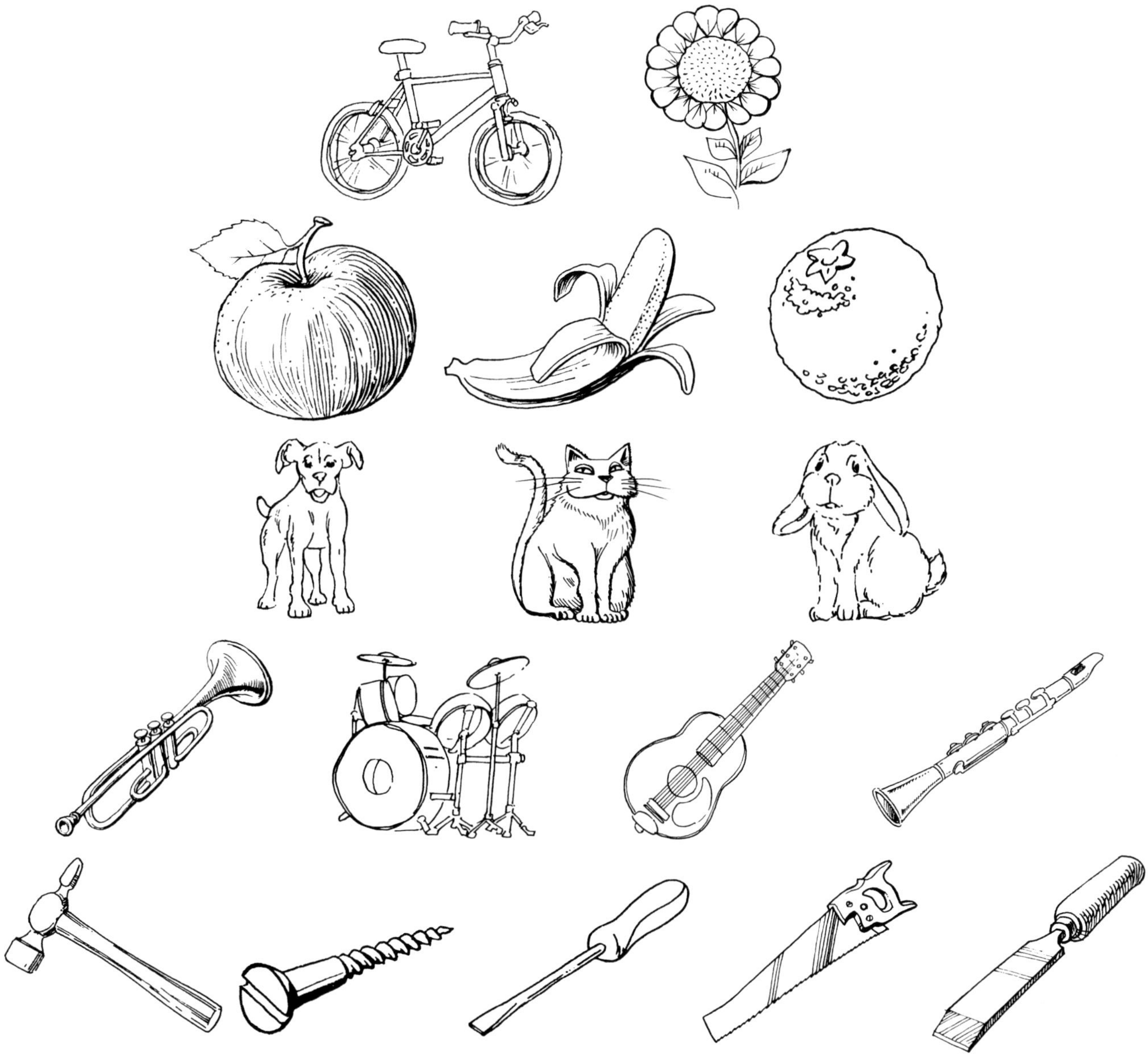

What strategies did you use?

How did you find this exercise? Easy ☐ OK ☐ Quite difficult ☐ Very difficult ☐

Remembering the design

How difficult do you think you will find this exercise? Easy ☐ OK ☐ Quite difficult ☐ Very difficult ☐

Instruction

Below are a number of designs drawn on a 9-dot matrix. Look at the top design for 60 seconds, and then cover it up by folding the piece of paper, or putting something over it. Now draw what you remember of the design on the 9-dot matrix provided. Repeat this for each of the designs and then make up your own designs and remember them using a strategy. The key to this exercise is to have a strategy for remembering the designs. Don't just see them as 15 individual lines, but rather as letters of the alphabet, words or shapes.

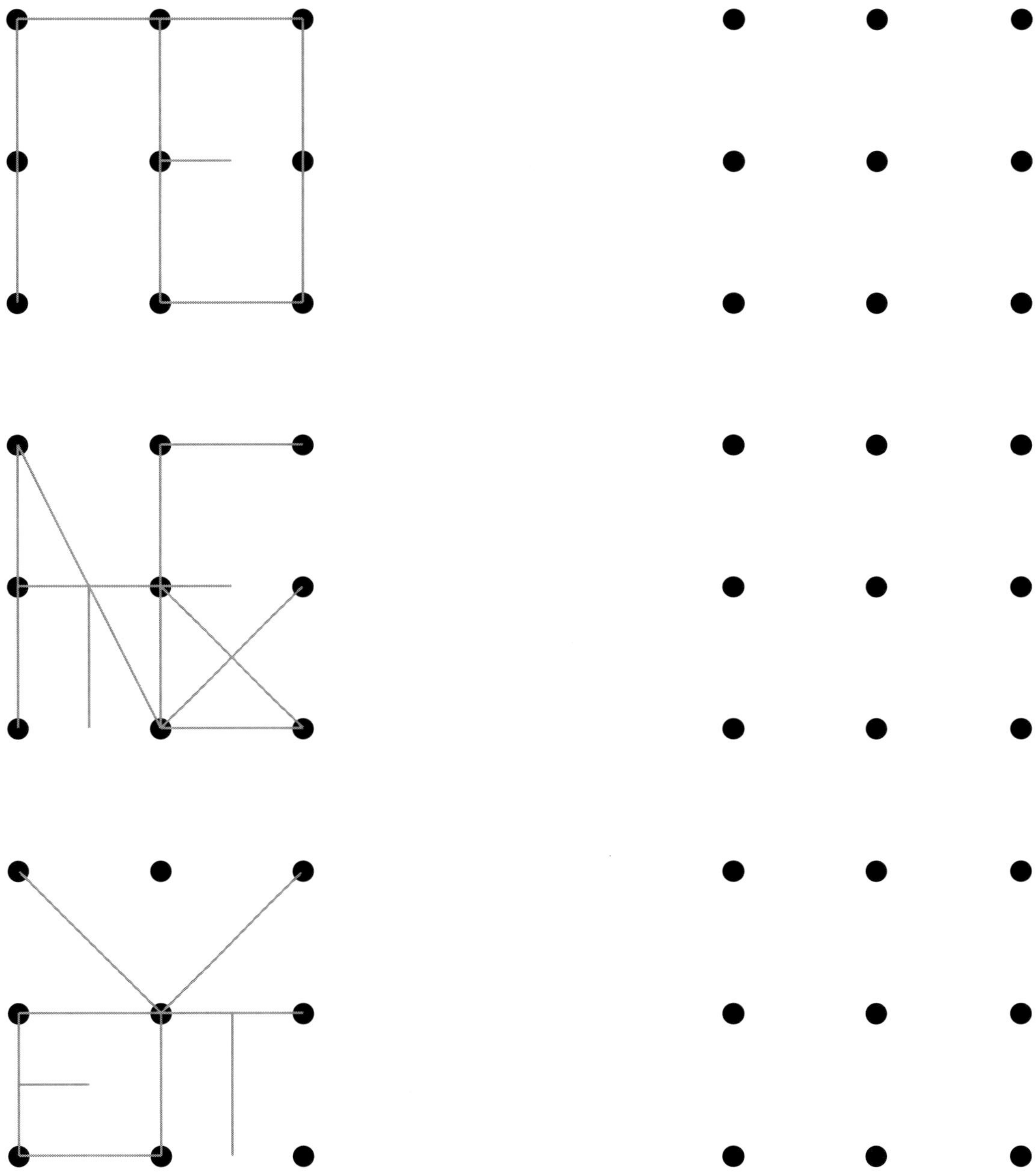

How did you find this exercise? Easy ☐ OK ☐ Quite difficult ☐ Very difficult ☐

EXERCISE 18

Stare at a person

How difficult do you think you will find this exercise? Easy ☐ OK ☐ Quite difficult ☐ Very difficult ☐

Instruction

You have one minute to look at a person very closely, and then you have to recall as many details as possible about that person's appearance. Either turn to the person next to you in the group, or carry out the activity with your therapist/family member. If you are working on your own, look at a picture.

When observing the person, use a strategy such as 'chunking' information into groups (eg, face, body, and clothes), or working from top to bottom. The point of the exercise is to remember as many details as possible. When the minute is up turn away from the person, and sit back to back. Now write down all of the details you can remember about that person's appearance. For each item you remember, you receive one point.

Write down everything you remember.

What strategies did you use to remember? What other strategies could you use?

How did you find this exercise? Easy ☐ OK ☐ Quite difficult ☐ Very difficult ☐

EXERCISE 19

Nine pictures – random memory task 1

How difficult do you think you will find this exercise? Easy ☐ OK ☐ Quite difficult ☐ Very difficult ☐

Instruction

Look at the pictures below and think of a way of remembering them. Decide which strategy to use. For instance, you could use 'chunking', 'grouping' (putting them together in groups), 'making an association', or 'making a story' using all the items. There are other strategies you can use too. You choose the strategy.

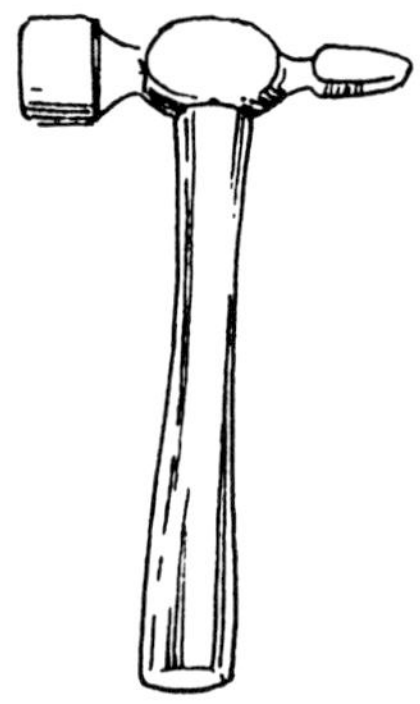
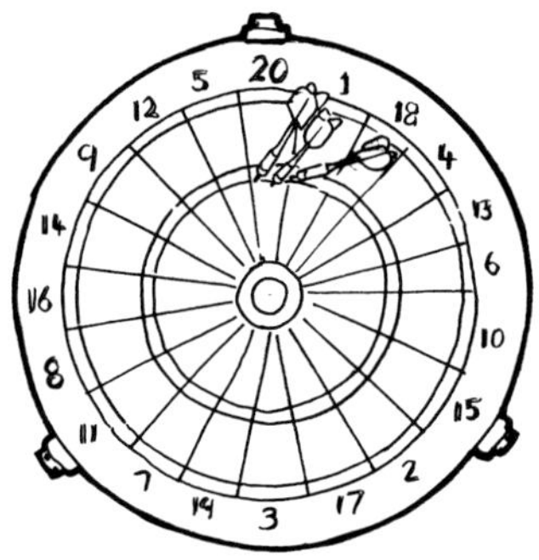
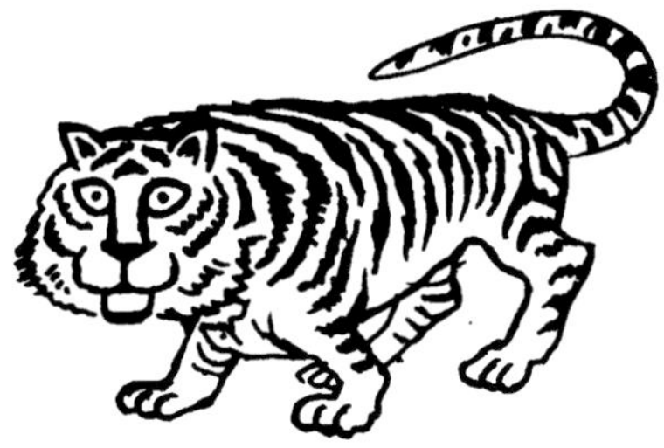
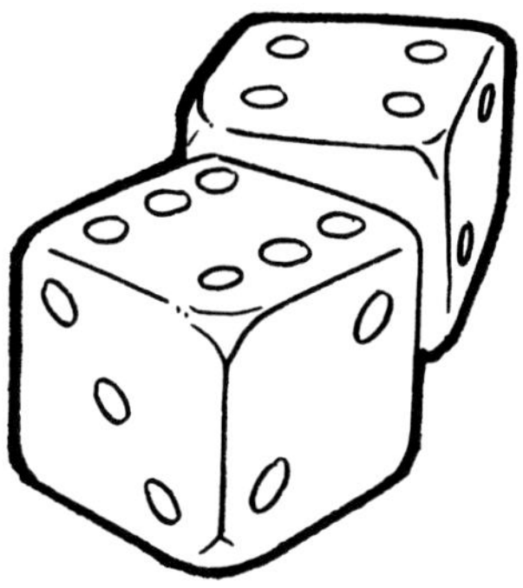
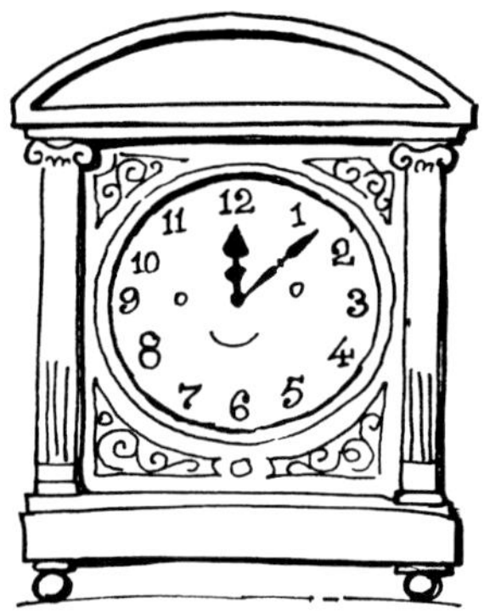
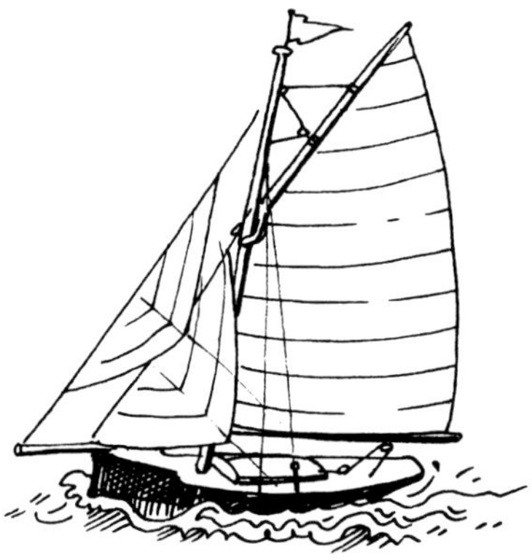
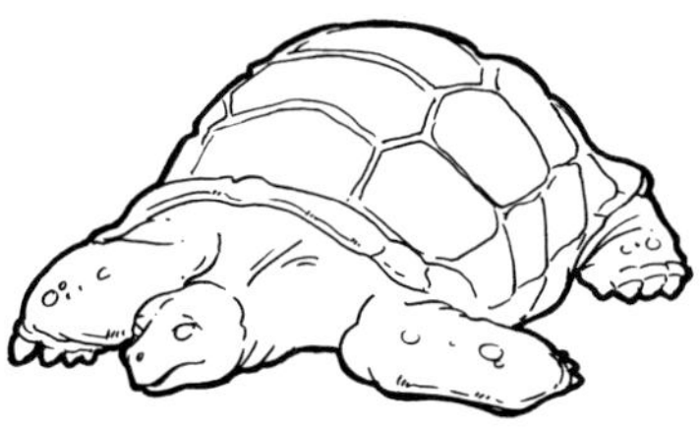
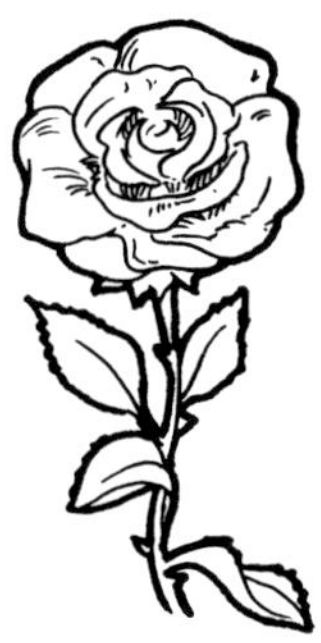
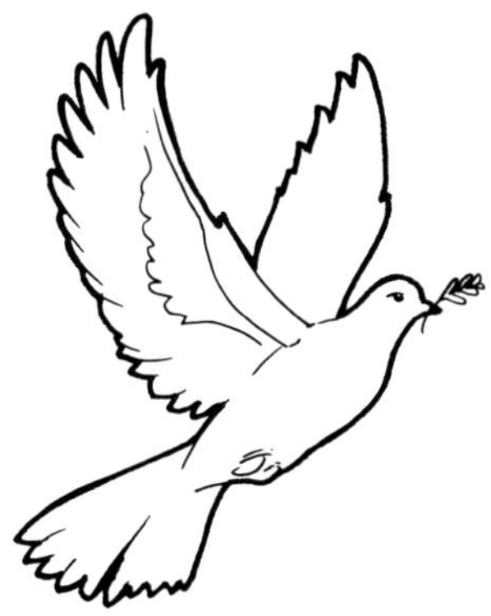

What strategies did you use?

How did you find this exercise? Easy ☐ OK ☐ Quite difficult ☐ Very difficult ☐

Chinese take-away

How difficult do you think you will find this exercise? Easy ☐ OK ☐ Quite difficult ☐ Very difficult ☐

Instruction

Look at the menu below, and order 10 items for a family of five. Use any strategy to remember (chunking, peg mnemonic, spider diagram, etc). Test your memory of the items after a delay of 30 minutes.

APPETISERS

1	Crispy Seaweed	£2.70
2	Barbecued Spare Ribs (Dry)	£3.25
3	Barbecued Spare Ribs with Peking Sauce	£3.25
4	Barbecued Spare Ribs with Salt & Spices	£3.25
5	Sesame Prawns on Toast	£3.25
6	Spring Roll	£1.60
7	Satay Chicken (S) (N)	£3.25
8	Cheese and Crabmeat Won Tons	£2.70
9	Quarter Crispy Duck with Pancakes	£6.95
15	Prawn Crackers	£1.30
15a	Crispy Won Ton with Sweet & Sour Sauce	£2.70

SOUP

16	Won Ton Soup	£2.20
17	Hot & Sour Soup	£2.20
18	Crab Meat Sweet Corn Soup	£1.80
19	Chicken Sweet Corn Soup	£1.80
20	Vegetable Soup	£1.80
21	Chicken Mushroom soup	£1.80

PORK DISHES

56	Sweet & Sour Pork	£4.00
57	Char Chiu (Barbequed Pork)	£4.00
58	Char Chiu with Vegetables	£4.00
58a	Special Chop Suey (Pork, Chicken, Prawn)	£4.25
59	Char Chiu with Asparagus	£4.00
60	Roast Pork in Spicy Sauce (S)	£4.00

CHICKEN DISHES

39	Grilled Chicken with Garlic Sauce	£4.00
40	Sweet & Sour Chicken	£4.00
41	Chicken with Pineapple	£4.00
42	Chicken with Black Bean & Green Peppers (S) (N)	£4.00
43	Chicken with Cashew Nuts (N)	£4.00
44	Chicken Curry (S) (N)	£4.00
55	Chicken Chop Suey	£4.00

BEEF DISHES

61	Beef with Mushrooms	£4.20
62	Sirloin Steak with Ginger & Spring Onions	£4.80
63	Sirloin Steak with Black Peppers (S)	£4.80
68	Crispy Shredded Beef with Chilli (S)	£4.80
69	Beef Curry (N)	£4.20
69a	Beef Chop Suey	£4.20

SEAFOOD DISHES

22	Deep Fried Squid in Salt & Chilli (S)	£4.00
23	Squid in Black Bean Sauce (S) (N)	£4.00
24	Squid Stir Fried with Asparagus	£4.00

NOODLES

78	Singapore Spicy Hot Vermicelli	£3.80
79	Crispy Noodles Fried with King Prawns	£4.50
80	Crispy Noodles Fried with Barbecued Pork	£3.50

VEGETABLE DISHES

92	Red Cooked Bean Curd	£3.20
93	Monks Mixed Vegetables with Bean Curd	£3.20
94	Stir Fried Mixed Vegetables	£3.20

PRAWN DISHES

25	Grilled King Prawn in Tomato Sauce	£4.50
26	Sweet & Sour Prawns	£4.50
27	Special Curry (Chicken, Prawn & Pork) (N)	£4.25
28	Stir Fried Prawns with Cashew Nuts (N)	£4.50
29	Stir Fried King Prawns in Black Bean and Green Pepper	£4.50
38a	King Prawn Chop Suey	£4.50

RICE DISHES

86	Special Fried Rice	£3.80
87	King Prawn Fried Rice	£4.50
88	Chicken Fried Rice	£3.50
89	Beef Fried Rice	£3.50
90	Egg Fried Rice	£1.90
91	Boiled Rice	£1.80

ENGLISH DISHES

102	King Prawn Omelette & Chips	£4.50
103	Chicken Omelette & Chips	£3.50
104	Mushrooms Omelette & Chips	£3.30
104a	Pork Chop with Chips & Curry Sauce	£4.80
104b	Chicken Fillet with Chips & Curry Sauce	£4.80

What strategy did you use to remember the 10 items?

How did you find this exercise? Easy ☐ OK ☐ Quite difficult ☐ Very difficult ☐

EXERCISE 21

Story-telling

How difficult do you think you will find this exercise? Easy ☐ OK ☐ Quite difficult ☐ Very difficult ☐

Instruction

Most people find it easier to remember a story than a series of unrelated words. So if you need to remember a number of items and can make them into a story you have a better chance of remembering. Practise using the storytelling strategy by making a story for the following lists and see if you can recall the items in 30 minutes' time:

1 You have been invited to dinner and need to take the following items:
- a bottle of wine
- a dessert
- candles

2 You need to buy the following items from the DIY store:
- nails
- a hammer
- light bulbs
- white emulsion paint

3 You are speaking at a council meeting tomorrow evening and want to make sure you cover the following points in your talk:
- abandoned cars
- parking permits
- rubbish collection
- an adventure playground in the park
- date of the next election

What strategy did you use to remember the items?

How did you find this exercise? Easy ☐ OK ☐ Quite difficult ☐ Very difficult ☐

Remembering a number

How difficult do you think you will find this exercise? Easy ☐ OK ☐ Quite difficult ☐ Very difficult ☐

Instruction

There appear to be more and more numbers to remember in everyday life – telephone numbers, PIN numbers, burglar alarm numbers, and car registration numbers. How do we remember them all?

There are a number of basic strategies, which may aid recall:

- **Chunking.** Break the number into chunks or sections. For example the phone number 9296471, becomes (9), as all numbers in this town start with that, then (296), and then the extension, which is (471).
- **Using a rhythm.** Add music to the number. If you can make the number more 'singalong', sometimes you can hear it in your head.
- **Making a sentence.** Translate the first nine digits into letters of the alphabet, and then make an appropriate sentence to remember the number. For example, if my PIN number were 9134, 9=I, 1=A, 3=C, 4=D. The sentence could be 'I am cash dispenser.'
- **Imagining the pattern.** If you have to press number keys, it is sometimes easier to remember the pattern or movement of your fingers rather than the number.
- **Storing securely.** Store numbers in an address book or mobile phone.
- **Personalising your PIN number.** Have all your PIN numbers the same, or the date of your birthday.

Task 1: What strategies do you use to remember important numbers?

Task 2: The registration number for my new car is P919 HGM. One way of remembering the number is the mnemonic P = Police, 919 (not quite 999); H = Have; G = Got; M = Me. See if you can remember this registration number 30 minutes later, using this strategy.

Task 3: Identify an important number that you would like to remember, and work out a way of remembering it.

How did you find this exercise? Easy ☐ OK ☐ Quite difficult ☐ Very difficult ☐

Using memory aids

How difficult do you think you will find this exercise? Easy ☐ OK ☐ Quite difficult ☐ Very difficult ☐

Instruction

We all use memory aids to some extent, but if you have had a brain injury it is more important to use them. What memory aids do you use?

		Always	Sometimes	Never
1	Do you carry a diary or notebook, and a pen or pencil with you?			
2	Do you keep a diary for appointments or fill in a diary describing events of the day?			
3	Do you use sticky labels to write lists and reminders?			
4	Do you plan your day by writing a list?			
5	Do you have a calendar on the wall at home where you can write in appointments and special events?			
6	Do you have a filing system at home for household bills?			
7	Do you have a special key hook at home, or a special place where you put your keys?			
8	Do you have an answering machine, or call minder system on your telephone at home?			
9	Do you make a shopping list before you go shopping?			
10	Do you have an address book, or filofax with an address section?			

What other memory aids do you use?

What is the most useful memory aid that you use?

How did you find this exercise? Easy ☐ OK ☐ Quite difficult ☐ Very difficult ☐

Thinking Skills

INFORMATION SHEETS

THINKING SKILLS EXERCISES

Thinking skills questionnaire

Name ______________________ Date ______________

Read each statement,and mark the box that best describes your behaviour now. It might be helpful to ask someone who knows you well to complete the questionnaire and fill in the independent scorer column.

Scoring Agree = 2 Partially agree = 1 Disagree = 0

Question	Score					
	Self-score			Independent scorer		
	Agree	Partially agree	Disagree	Agree Agree	Partially agree	Disagree
General thinking skills – information processing **1** It takes me longer to think – my speed is slower.						
2 I sometimes get confused or overloaded when there is a lot going on.						
3 My thinking is less subtle or flexible, and tends to be more concrete, rigid, and black and white.						
Thinking score. *(All the exercises (1–28) should be of benefit.)*						
Attention skills **1** I find it hard to concentrate for long periods of time, and get distracted easily.						
2 I find it more difficult to filter out background noise.						
3 I have problems doing more than one thing at the same time – dividing or switching my attention.						
Attention score. *(Pay particular attention to Exercises 19–28.)*						
Language skills **1** I sometimes have problems finding the right word.						
2 I have problems understanding or taking in the speech of others.						
3 My conversation is less fluent and precise and sometimes I have difficulty 'getting to the point'.						
Language score. *(Pay particular attention to Exercises 1–16.)*						
Perceptual and visuo-spatial skills **1** I have difficulty judging distances and being aware of space.						
2 I have greater difficulty putting shapes or mechanical things together.						
3 I sometimes miss things on the edges of my visual field.						
Perceptual score. *(Pay particular attention to Exercises 17 and 18.)*						

How relevant did you find this sheet? Very ☐ Slightly ☐ Not very ☐

Thinking skills: what are they?

This section concentrates on a cluster of skills that, for convenience, we will call thinking skills. It does not include memory and executive skills, although in real life all these cognitive skills are closely connected and interlinked. Thinking skills have a number of key features:

Attention is a key cognitive skill – the basis of all new learning and memory; a vital component of executive ability, and a skill that underpins all recovery and rehabilitation after brain injury. People with attention problems often say that they can no longer concentrate on reading books, or having multiple conversations; or they might say that they have difficulty studying for any length of time. There are different types of attention:

- *Sustained attention* refers to concentrating for prolonged periods of time on the same thing, such as studying, watching television, or reading. People with problems in this area often say that their 'minds drift off', or they get distracted and end up thinking of something else.
- *Selective attention* involves selecting one aspect of our environment and ignoring or filtering out all the background noise, or other distractions. After brain injury, people often say that they are unable to filter out irrelevant distractions.
- *Divided attention* is the ability to pay attention to two or more things at the same time. One student found it difficult to listen to what the teacher was saying and take notes at the same time. This skill demands the ability to switch attention very rapidly from one source to another.

Information-processing refers to our ability to make sense of the information that pours into our brains via our attention and sensory mechanisms. This involves many different skills, including:

- *Speed of thinking* is the rate at which information can be taken in, processed and then acted upon – 'how fast the cogs turn'.
- *Capacity of thinking* is the amount of information that can be taken in during any one sitting – whether you're 'firing on all four cylinders'.
- *Abstracting* is the ability to think in an abstract, non-concrete way: to think of something without it being placed right in front of you, and to make links between different things or events.
- *Organisation skills* are the many different ways in which the brain organises information, including matching, discriminating, sequencing, grouping, categorising and ordering.

Thinking skills: what are they?

Sensory and perceptual skills are the skills we use to interpret our world – or the information that our senses (vision, smell, touch, and sound) have brought into our brains. Our eyes might see and our nose might smell, but it is the part of the brain that processes, or makes sense of that information, that is vitally important. People with perceptual problems sometimes think there is something wrong with their eyesight; but an eye test shows there is nothing wrong. This problem is with the brain, not the eyes.

Language skills involve both receptive ability – understanding streams of words strung together in sentences by others – and expressive ability – putting words together to make your own sentences. Often after a brain injury, people say they have greater difficulty finding the right word. They might say 'the word is on the tip of my tongue', or 'I know what it is, but I can't find the right word.'

Conscious and automatic processing
As we become familiar with a task it becomes automatic to us (eg, driving). While we learn a new task we often have to consciously think about it, but as we develop skill at that task we seem to carry it out automatically. This frees up our attention capacity, so we can focus it on other novel tasks and situations. Once we become proficient at driving a car we can drive and listen to the radio or have a conversation at the same time. If this movement from conscious to automatic did not happen, then we would quickly become overloaded by the demands of life. Following brain injury, it seems that many of those skills that functioned on an automatic level now operate at a conscious level – more slowly and with more effort. So after brain injury, many people reach a point of information overload much earlier than they would have done before their injury.

1 Name three different kinds of attention.
2 List the different skills that make up information-processing.
3 Explain the concept of automatic and conscious processing. Why is this an important concept to understand?

How relevant did you find this sheet? Very ☐ Slightly ☐ Not very ☐

Ways of improving attention and concentration

- **Engage in stimulating activity for gradually extended periods of time**. Focused active stimulation, which involves multiple brain cells firing, is helpful. Activities that require active rather than passive thinking are best. Watching television is not such an active process as trying to solve a problem.

- **Minimise distractions**. Try to work in a quiet environment with no background distractions, such as noisy televisions or people talking. Let people know they should try not to interrupt you when you are working.

- **Take frequent breaks**. If the problem is made worse by fatigue, work for shorter periods of time and take breaks. The student who works a little and often, perhaps for periods of up to 30 minutes, is likely to be more productive.

- **Talk to yourself – say things out loud**. By simply saying, 'What should I be doing now?', or 'Stay focused', or reading instructions out loud, you can help yourself to stay on the right track.

- **Use environmental cueing**. Have a cue card in your work area with a simple message on it, such as 'Focus on what to do'. This can often help you to avoid drifting off. You could also try wearing a digital watch that bleeps every 20 minutes or so, which acts as a cue to stay focused or to check your work.

- **Set yourself targets or goals**. Having something definite to work towards will help you stay motivated. If you find you are achieving it too easily, then set yourself harder targets.

- **Use incentives**. When you achieve a target or goal reward yourself. Try something very simple, such as a cup of tea or coffee, or a biscuit; letting yourself watch a TV programme, or going for a walk.

- **Gain control – be assertive**. If in everyday conversation you feel you are being overloaded and you cannot attend to all the information, request that the person slows down their delivery or repeats himself. Be assertive, and say something like, 'Excuse me, I think you have lost me, could you repeat that?'.

- **Best time**. Work out when your best time of day is for doing this kind of work. Try to set up your daily schedule to take account of this. Most people find it best to work in the mornings.

Ways of improving attention and concentration

- **One thing at a time**. Concentrate on one thing at a time. Do not try to take in too much information at once, as this leads to mistakes. Do one thing, then move on to the next.

- **Don't rush things**. You may find you have a tendency to rush everyday tasks and end up making mistakes. Take your time, and pace yourself.

- **Apply structure**. Whenever possible, make a plan, keep a record, or break things down into manageable parts. If you do get distracted, you can easily pick up where you left off.

- **Self monitor or check and double-check your work**. Do this with everything you do. It will be slow and hard at first, but it will become a habit as you get accustomed to it. This is the only sure-fire way of picking up on your own errors.

> **1** Which strategies do you actually use in everyday life at the moment to help you concentrate?
> **2** Identify three of the strategies described that you think could improve your concentration.

How relevant did you find this sheet? Very ☐ Slightly ☐ Not very ☐

Ways of improving language skills

Problems with language are often referred to as 'aphasia' and can be broken down into two areas. First, *expressive aphasia* – using language to express ideas and thoughts. This is a complex skill that involves selecting the right word, and then making the correct sound. Second *receptive aphasia* – the ability to understand the speech of others. This can vary from mild receptive aphasia, when you are less able to understand complex sentence formations, to severe receptive aphasia, when you do not understand language at all.

Coping with word-finding difficulties

- When searching for the name of an object, describe it, talk around it; do not get hung up on finding the exact right word. Remember that it is getting the message across which matters, not getting the word or sound exactly right.

- When trying to retrieve a word, search your memory in an organised way, going through different categories and sub-categories. For example, when trying to think of a person's name, ask yourself questions, such as, 'Is the person male?' Then go through letters of the alphabet.

- Use gestures and signs associated with a particular word if you cannot access exactly that word.

Helping people who have a language difficulty

- Do not speak very quickly, and try to use short sentences with familiar words.

- Try not to jump from one topic to another in conversation.

- Reduce background noise and other distractions.

- Do not pressurise the person, insisting that they say the word, and resist the temptation to speak for them or finish their sentences.

- Do not pretend that you understand if you do not. Try not to patronise: remember you are dealing with an intelligent adult.

- If you understand a part of what the person said, repeat those words, so that they do not have to go through it all again, and provide a prompt. For example, 'You say you went on holiday where?'

1 Identify one way of trying to recall a person's name if you can't think of it.
2 Identify two strategies to help communicate with a person who has a significant word-finding difficulty.

How relevant did you find this sheet? Very ☐ Slightly ☐ Not very ☐

Understanding and coping with perceptual and visuo-spatial difficulties

These are a group of skills that we use to make sense of the world we perceive. They mainly involve a part of the brain that processes information coming in through the eyes or any other sense organ. Visual processing tends to be in the areas known as the parietal and occipital lobes, at the back of the brain. Some people suffer from a condition called visual neglect, where they do not perceive what is in their peripheral visual field. Other people might have difficulty judging distances, reading maps, recognising objects or shapes, putting mechanical or technical things together, or with any task that involves visuo-spatial or perceptual skills.

Improving perceptual skills

- Scanning. Move your head slightly; look to the left, and look to the right. This helps you to process information at the periphery of your visual field.
- Use written and visual cues.
- If you have a left-sided visual neglect, the simple act of moving your left hand and arm up and down for about an hour a week improves your functioning. This is because the physical activity of moving your arm reactivates neural circuits in the area involved with visuo-spatial ability.
- Practise copying complex shapes, such as cubes or stars; bisecting lines in the middle; doing puzzles and jigsaws, or any task that involves identifying shapes.

1 What area of the brain is involved with perception and visuo-spatial ability?
2 If you have a left-sided visual neglect, and tend to ignore things on the left side, what strategies can you use to improve this?

How relevant did you find this sheet? Very ☐ Slightly ☐ Not very ☐

Thinking skills quiz

1 Why is attention such an important cognitive skill?

2 Describe three different kinds of attention.

3 Describe three different strategies for improving your attention and concentration.

4 Explain why, even if your eyesight is fine, you may have problems identifying or copying a complex shape.

5 If somebody has a problem understanding or receiving language, identify two things that you could do in your speech to help.

How relevant did you find this sheet? Very ☐ Slightly ☐ Not very ☐

EXERCISE 1

Synonyms

How difficult do you think you will find this exercise? Easy ☐ OK ☐ Quite difficult ☐ Very difficult ☐

Instruction

Look at each of the words, and write down two other words that mean the same or a similar thing.

Home			Attack		
Stool			Relax		
Boat			Curtains		
Family			Club		
Drink			Toilet		
Plant			Bonnet		
Rug			Embrace		
Ship			Excited		
Attractive			Smash		
Explode			Fall		
Plant			Smile		
Ecstatic			Drunk		

Think of a word of your own, and then think of two other words that have the same or similar meanings.
Try to make the words as hard as possible.

Identify any useful strategy for helping you think of words.

How did you find this exercise? Easy ☐ OK ☐ Quite difficult ☐ Very difficult ☐

EXERCISE 2

Antonyms

How difficult do you think you will find this exercise? Easy ☐ OK ☐ Quite difficult ☐ Very difficult ☐

Instruction

Look at each of the words, and write down two other words that have the opposite meaning.

Sad			Help		
Soft			Valley		
Attractive			Complex		
Warm			Deep		
Courageous			Curve		
Easy			Beg		
Colourful			Congratulate		
Smart			Scrutinise		
Tall			Scrape		
Expensive			Block		
Dance			Shuffle		
Forget			Blow		

Think of a word of your own, and then think of two other words that have opposite meanings.
Try to make the words as hard as possible.

Identify any useful strategy for helping you think of words

How did you find this exercise? Easy ☐ OK ☐ Quite difficult ☐ Very difficult ☐

Rearrange the sentence

How difficult do you think you will find this exercise? Easy ☐ OK ☐ Quite difficult ☐ Very difficult ☐

Instruction

Rearrange the scrambled words on each line to make a sentence. Write the words on the line, or say them out loud. Do not leave out any words.

1 cats milk like

____

2 bag my was heavy

____

3 painting very was the beautiful

____

4 the take to car I must my garage

____

5 late running is the ten minutes train

____

6 wines produce quality French the high

____

7 the day stopped all ringing phone has not

____

Now try to make up your own scrambled sentence that says something about you.

How did you find this exercise? Easy ☐ OK ☐ Quite difficult ☐ Very difficult ☐

EXERCISE 4

Word association

How difficult do you think you will find this exercise? Easy ☐ OK ☐ Quite difficult ☐ Very difficult ☐

Instruction

Read the three words on each line, and think of an object – a noun – that those words describe. For example: sharp, metal, lunch = knife.

- ➤ Roll, sticky, clear =
- ➤ Wrinkles, steam, clothes =
- ➤ Feathers, black, fly =
- ➤ Border, wood, post =
- ➤ Stripe, hooves, crossing =
- ➤ Metal, paper, cuts =
- ➤ Exhaust, ticket, travel =
- ➤ Wallet, plastic, signature =
- ➤ Clothes, wet, peg =
- ➤ Green, iron, card =
- ➤ Light, bulb, pavement =
- ➤ Warm, water, pipe =
- ➤ Hard, black, playtime =
- ➤ Sugar, tin, rise =
- ➤ Blade, wood, adjust =
- ➤ Round, hole, cotton =
- ➤ Soft, nose, pocket =
- ➤ Water, visibility, mountain-top =
- ➤ Pump, body, love =
- ➤ Hot, space, god =

Now try to make up your own word associations and try it out on the group.

How did you find this exercise? Easy ☐ OK ☐ Quite difficult ☐ Very difficult ☐

The right word

How difficult do you think you will find this exercise? Easy ☐ OK ☐ Quite difficult ☐ Very difficult ☐

Instruction

Below is a list of words. For each individual key word, think of a one-word clue that will help your partner or the group members guess what the key word is. If they do not guess on the first word clue, you have to provide a second word clue. If they still have not guessed correctly, give them a third word clue.

For example: The original key word is 'tomato'. The first clue could be 'salad' or even better 'ketchup'. The second clue might be 'red', etc.

This exercise can be carried out alone or in a group. In a group, hand out the words on cards and ask the whole group to help guess what the word is.

Key word	first clue	second clue	third clue
Train			
Carrot			
Tie			
Broom			
Table			
Atlas			
Kitten			
Mountain			
Swan			
Grapefruit			
Ruler			
Street lamp			
Milk			
Wrist-watch			
Frog			
Football			
Wine			
Newspaper			
Battle of Hastings			
Boxing glove			
Needle			
The Beatles			
Golf ball			
Prime Minister			
The Bible			
London			
Referee			
A medal			
Curry			
Wallpaper			

How did you find this exercise? Easy ☐ OK ☐ Quite difficult ☐ Very difficult ☐

Words with multiple meanings

How difficult do you think you will find this exercise? Easy ☐ OK ☐ Quite difficult ☐ Very difficult ☐

Instruction

Give two or more meanings for the following words. Do not worry about the spelling – you are only thinking about the phonetic sound.

For example: DRAFT. The first meaning could be 'a wind'. The second meaning could be 'a first version of a written document'. The third meaning could be 'to be conscripted into the armed services'.

The spelling of each given word may be altered as long as they sound the same. Note: There is not always a third meaning for each of these words.

Word	**First meaning**	**Second meaning**	**Third meaning**
Spring			
Blue			
Through			
Plant			
Right			
Table			
Nail			
Bean			
Marble			
Step			
Grass			
Bat			
Train			
Score			
Prize			
Court			
Stick			

Now try to think of other words with multiple meanings.

How did you find this exercise? Easy ☐ OK ☐ Quite difficult ☐ Very difficult ☐

EXERCISE 7

Analogies

How difficult do you think you will find this exercise? Easy ☐ OK ☐ Quite difficult ☐ Very difficult ☐

Instruction

Complete the following analogies.

For example: Lead is to heavy as Feather is to light.

- Shoe is to foot as Glove is to ____________________
- Lion is to jungle as Bat is to ____________________
- Mechanic is to car as Plumber is to ____________________
- Banana is to peel as Bread is to ____________________
- Referee is to soccer as Umpire is to ____________________
- Nail polish is to nail as Mascara is to ____________________
- Gun is to bullet as Hose is to ____________________
- Hair is to wig as Teeth are to ____________________
- Ant is to nest as Bees are to ____________________
- Heart is to chest as Brain is to ____________________
- Guitar is to string as Piano is to ____________________
- Watch is to strap as Trousers are to ____________________
- January is to winter as September is to ____________________
- The Koran is to Muslims as the Bible is to ____________________
- Cake is to baking as Carrots are to ____________________
- Driver is to car as Pilot is to ____________________
- General is to Army as Admiral is to ____________________

Now try to make up your own analogies.

How did you find this exercise? Easy ☐ OK ☐ Quite difficult ☐ Very difficult ☐

EXERCISE 8

Odd one out

How difficult do you think you will find this exercise? Easy ☐ OK ☐ Quite difficult ☐ Very difficult ☐

Instruction
In each row, circle the item that is the odd one out.

5	7	2	1	9	3
Jack	Jane	John	Pete	Mike	Dave
Oak	Chestnut	Pine	Willow	Poplar	Beech
Sheep	Cow	Horse	Rabbit	Kangaroo	Goat
Thailand	Mexico	Egypt	New York	Canada	Italy
Violin	Banjo	Guitar	Cello	Harp	Oboe
Bat	Flag	Ball	Green	Tee	Club
Mouse	Rat	Keyboard	Disc	Icon	Hard drive
Brush	Canvas	Frame	Paint	Gallery	Jewel
Cola	Cookie	Bread	Porridge	Cereal	Oat Cake
Glass	Mug	Teacup	Saucer	Flask	Bottle
Gun	Knife	Poison	Cheque	Spear	Sword
Tie	Tiara	Crown	Necklace	Brooch	Ring
Ham	Pork	Trotters	Chicken	Bacon	Gammon
Car	Bicycle	Truck	Van	Bus	Ambulance

Now make up your own list of words with one odd one for each row. Give this list to someone else to see if they can guess which is your 'odd' word.

How did you find this exercise? Easy ☐ OK ☐ Quite difficult ☐ Very difficult ☐

Complete the word

How difficult do you think you will find this exercise? Easy ☐ OK ☐ Quite difficult ☐ Very difficult ☐

Instruction

In the list below, complete the word. The letters given might be the beginning, end or middle of a word. There is a clue in the column on the right.

For example:

NEL = KENNEL (Home for pet)

ENT		Way in
PUR		Colour
GIN		Start
MAN		City
PAT		Design
BAL		Vote
OPP		Completely different
NER		Worried
SET		Calm
BAD		Sport
USH		Used for painting
SON		An individual
LET		Ladies' room
EST		Search
NER		Bend
ENC		Something to write with
PHA		Big animal
BET		Group of letters

Now make up your own part words, and try them out on the group.

How did you find this exercise? Easy ☐ OK ☐ Quite difficult ☐ Very difficult ☐

Connections

How difficult do you think you will find this exercise? Easy ☐ OK ☐ Quite difficult ☐ Very difficult ☐

Instruction

Starting with a word in the column on the left, think of three associations or connections to reach the word in the column on the right.

For example:

Starting word = Tree, and final word = Jellyfish.
Tree – Christmas tree – Holiday – Jellyfish

Cat			A tissue
Grass			A murder
A tin of tuna			A party dress
One sock			House
A tie			Soccer
A dead mouse			Shed
Car			Oasis
A knife			Farm
Tony Blair			Wig
A postman			Suicide

Now work out your own connections, and try them out on other people.

How did you find this exercise? Easy ☐ OK ☐ Quite difficult ☐ Very difficult ☐

Proverbs 1

How difficult do you think you will find this exercise? Easy ☐ OK ☐ Quite difficult ☐ Very difficult ☐

Instruction

Describe in your own words what each of the proverbs means.

- Make hay while the sun shines.
- Two's company, three's a crowd.
- Leave no stone unturned.
- No man is an island.
- Rome was not built in a day.
- The pot calling the kettle black.
- A little knowledge is a dangerous thing.
- When the going gets tough the tough get going.
- Beggars can't be choosers.
- Out of sight, out of mind.
- Mighty oaks from little acorns grow.
- Don't cry over spilt milk.
- Many hands make light work.
- A picture is worth a thousand words.
- You can't see the wood for the trees.
- You can't teach an old dog new tricks.
- All that glitters is not gold.
- Practice makes perfect.
- All work and no play make Jack a dull boy.
- A bird in the hand is worth two in the bush.

Think of your own proverb or expression, and describe a situation in which it might be used.

How did you find this exercise? Easy ☐ OK ☐ Quite difficult ☐ Very difficult ☐

EXERCISE 12

Proverbs 2

How difficult do you think you will find this exercise? Easy ☐ OK ☐ Quite difficult ☐ Very difficult ☐

Instruction

Choose one of the expressions or proverbs and explain what it means to someone else in the group. You must do this without mentioning the key words that are underlined. The members of the group have to guess which expression or proverb you are describing. They can use the list to help them.

- Hit the nail on the head.
- Eats like a pig.
- Left a bad taste in my mouth.
- Birds of a feather flock together.
- A chip off the old block.
- Jack of all trades.
- Every cloud has a silver lining.
- Don't pass the buck.
- Beggars can't be choosers.
- Out of sight, out of mind.
- You're walking on thin ice.
- Don't make a mountain out of a molehill.
- It's like finding a needle in a haystack.
- It takes two to tango.
- Don't open a can of worms.
- The grass is always greener on the other side.
- A stitch in time saves nine.
- When in Rome, do as the Romans do.
- Don't beat around the bush.
- It's like getting blood out of a stone.

Think of another proverb or expression, and write it down. Give the group clues to guess what it is, without mentioning any of the key words in the expression.

How did you find this exercise? Easy ☐ OK ☐ Quite difficult ☐ Very difficult ☐

EXERCISE 13

Category breakdown

How difficult do you think you will find this exercise? Easy ☐ OK ☐ Quite difficult ☐ Very difficult ☐

Instruction

For each of the categories given below, write words that begin with the letter shown in the left column. You have one minute to do each category. Split the group into teams.

	Fruit and vegetables	Drinks	Countries	Animals
A				
C				

	Trees and plants	Cities	Cars	Jobs
B				
R				

Use any letter for these categories.

Things that are round	Things that are stripy	Things that cause pain	Things related to a wedding

How did you find this exercise? Easy ☐ OK ☐ Quite difficult ☐ Very difficult ☐

What's the question?

How difficult do you think you will find this exercise? Easy ☐ OK ☐ Quite difficult ☐ Very difficult ☐

Instruction

Work out the correct questions that give the answers listed below. The question you select must lead naturally to the following answer, with correct grammar and context.

Question	**Answer**
For example: Who wears a blue uniform and upholds the law?	A policeman
	A ruler
	Turnips
	Tony Blair
	A video recorder
	An aspirin
	A girl called Sarah
	The toilet
	Marmalade on toast
	Just south of Birmingham
	Yes, I saw him on Tuesday
	Half of 50
	The cheque is in the post
	When I retire

Now make up your own answers, and give them to the group to work out a possible question for each. Try to make them as difficult as possible.

Question	**Answer**

How did you find this exercise? Easy ☐ OK ☐ Quite difficult ☐ Very difficult ☐

Correct interpretation

How difficult do you think you will find this exercise? Easy ☐ OK ☐ Quite difficult ☐ Very difficult ☐

Instruction

Tick the rows in which the sentence is similar to the proverb and put a cross where it is not.

1	If you start early you will be rewarded.	The early bird catches the worm.	
2	When doing long jump or leaping, make sure you have the right footwear.	Look before you leap.	
3	If you are determined, you will succeed.	Where there's a will there's a way.	
4	Dad likes his son.	Like father, like son.	
5	It is good to be late.	Better late than never.	
6	If too many people are involved, they get in each other's way.	Too many cooks spoil the broth.	
7	Beware – cats are dangerous animals.	Curiosity killed the cat.	
8	If you do something for me, I will look after you.	One good turn deserves another.	
9	Take advantage of an opportunity when it presents itself.	Strike while the iron is hot.	
10	Every day watch out for something new to happen.	Don't count your chickens before they hatch.	
11	When one bad thing happens, another one follows close behind.	When it rains, it pours.	
12	If somebody does not have a job it means they are lazy.	Don't judge a book by its cover.	
13	People with similar interests usually do not get on very well.	Birds of a feather flock together.	
14	You have to crack an egg to make an omelette.	Don't put all of your eggs in one basket.	
15	After it rains it will be sunny very soon.	Every cloud has a silver lining.	
16	He gets to the point of the discussion or issue quickly.	He hits the nail on the head.	

Make up your own proverbs, with either correct or incorrect explanations.

17			
18			

How did you find this exercise? Easy ☐ OK ☐ Quite difficult ☐ Very difficult ☐

EXERCISE 16

Twenty questions

How difficult do you think you will find this exercise? Easy ☐ OK ☐ Quite difficult ☐ Very difficult ☐

Instruction

One person in the group thinks of an item or famous person, and everybody else in the group has to guess who or what it is by asking questions. The catch is that the group can only ask questions that can be answered by 'Yes' or 'No'. The aim of the exercise is to guess what the person is thinking, using as few questions as possible. A maximum of 20 questions may be asked before the group must guess who or what the person was thinking of. Each person in the group takes it in turn to think of an object or person. *Note:* the rest of the group must know the object or person.

Before starting, try these exercises.

1 Guessing a famous person

	If you were guessing a famous person, rank in order the questions you would ask to gain the most information. The first question has been provided as an example.
1	'Is this person male?'
2	
3	
4	
5	

2 Guessing an object: 'animal, vegetable or mineral'

	If you were guessing an object, rank in order the questions you would ask to gain the most information. The first two questions have been provided as an example.
1	'Is this thing an animal?'
2	'Is this thing a vegetable?'
3	
4	
5	

How did you find this exercise? Easy ☐ OK ☐ Quite difficult ☐ Very difficult ☐

Match the logos

How difficult do you think you will find this exercise? Easy ☐ OK ☐ Quite difficult ☐ Very difficult ☐

Instruction

Identify which company logos these sections are taken from. Look at the top set of company logos and bottom set of sections, and match them up.

1 The National Lottery

2 Levi's

3 Penguin Books

4 Ford

5 Paramount

6 Lego

7 Ikea

8 Adidas

9 Channel 4

10 Mercedes-Benz

11 Pepsi

12 Yellow pages

1 ____________

2 ____________

3 ____________

4 ____________

5 ____________

6 ____________

7 ____________

8 ____________

9 ____________

10 ____________

11 ____________

12 ____________

How did you find this exercise? Easy ☐ OK ☐ Quite difficult ☐ Very difficult ☐

Match the traffic signs

How difficult do you think you will find this exercise? Easy ☐ OK ☐ Quite difficult ☐ Very difficult ☐

Instruction

Identify which traffic signs these sections are taken from. Look at the top set of traffic signs and the bottom set of sections, and match them up.

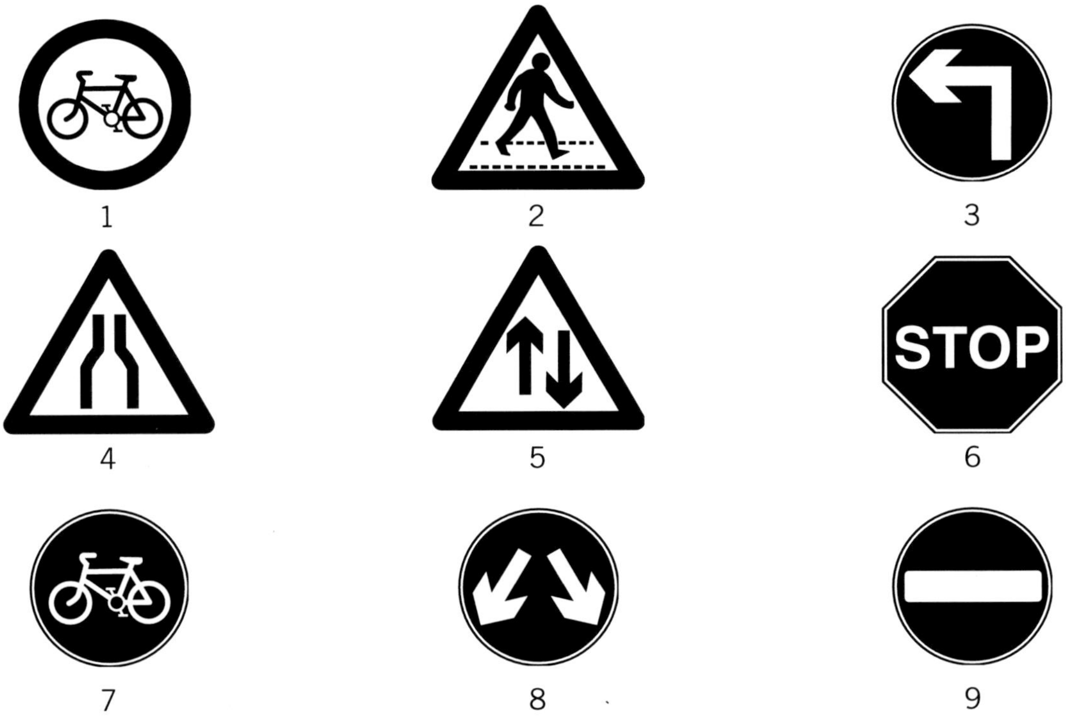

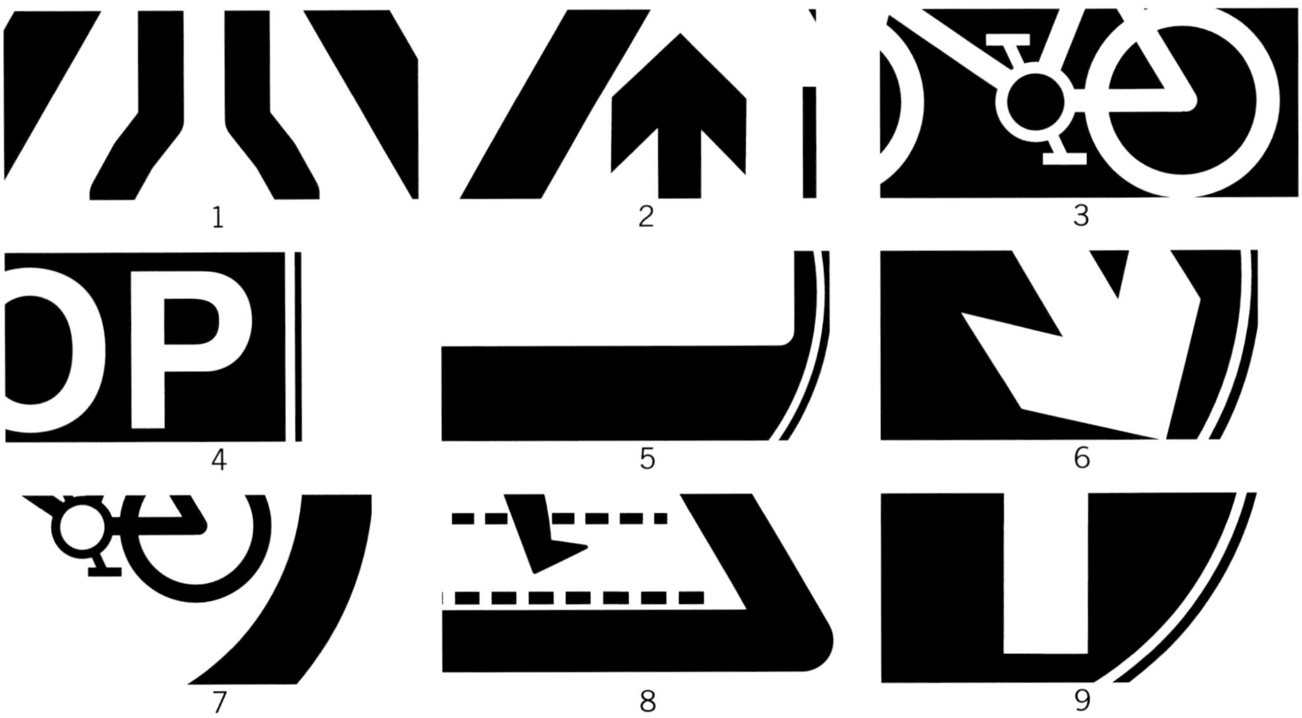

How did you find this exercise? Easy ☐ OK ☐ Quite difficult ☐ Very difficult ☐

Mental sorting

How difficult do you think you will find this exercise? Easy ☐ OK ☐ Quite difficult ☐ Very difficult ☐

Instruction

Read the categories next to each square, then put the items from the list into the correct categories on the grid. This is an exercise in dividing and switching attention and thinking of more than one thing at a time.

	I own	**I don't own**
Heavier than me		
Lighter than me		

horse pencil toothbrush television shoes trousers

slippers car watch compact disc hen tie

diamond ring dog bus computer caravan hair gel

	I can do at present	**I could not do at present**
Hobbies		
Jobs		

play football rock climbing fishing lawyer play golf

teacher scientist sales manager run a marathon

collect stamps milkman drive swim cinema

read a book cook a meal typist go to a gym

work in a garden centre

How did you find this exercise? Easy ☐ OK ☐ Quite difficult ☐ Very difficult ☐

Embedded words 1

How difficult do you think you will find this exercise? Easy ☐ OK ☐ Quite difficult ☐ Very difficult ☐

Instruction

This task aims to improve divided attention.

Look at the list and mark the words that refer to the following characteristics.

1 Circle 'stripy' words [ ], while at the same time single cross out 'food' words [ ].

2 Underline 'sticky' words [ ], while at the same time double cross out 'straight' words [ ].

3 Identify which words are mentioned twice. Add up the total in each category.

egg rose London sellotape® rock fish zebra music
tissue John cat glue bright super fly American flag
diamond star annual switch parrot witch dance
Velcro square kitchen lined paper computer holiday ice-
cream granite barcode pen grass blue four granite
rabbit pillow ruler swan chicken Roman road swerve
tennis crow bee radiator glass cold toffee mutton
mountain barber's pole silk Africa seaside hair
paperclip treacle port cola month triangle five
blanket bed silk London cloud paper water pie
maths subway pomp music fur piano keyboard pills
beef wallet wrist tiger clown jam milk watch
sand lake bridge kite kitten map balloon baboon
stick carrot hitch club light-rays broach wasp
diamond bath melted cheese French flag book goat
wallpaper paste square bag carrot flipper horizon
swimming sock deer brick laser beam hot tarmac worm
ant balloon swear kangaroo nice radio crash
underwear honey alphabet car sergeant's chevrons curry

What strategies did you use to complete this task?

How did you find this exercise? Easy ☐ OK ☐ Quite difficult ☐ Very difficult ☐

Embedded words 2

How difficult do you think you will find this exercise? Easy ☐ OK ☐ Quite difficult ☐ Very difficult ☐

Instruction

This task aims to improve divided attention.

Look at the list and mark the words that refer to the following characteristics.

1 Circle 'hot' words [ ], while at the same time single cross out 'animal' words [ ].

2 Underline 'musical' words [ ], while at the same time double cross out 'place-names' words [ ].

3 Identify which words are mentioned twice. Add up the total in each category.

fire	violin	Rome	sellotape®	rock	bear	zebra	sun	
tissue	one	cat	glue	brimstone	super	mouse		
American flag	diamond	York	switch	mole	witch	dance		
Velcro	three	kitchen	burn	computer	holiday	ice-cream		
note	barcode	pen	grass	blue	four	granite	rabbit	
pillow	ruler	hen	scald	Roman road	swerve	tennis		
wolf	flame	glass	Canada	toffee	lamb	mountain		
barber's pole	sun	Africa	sea	drum	paperclip	treacle		
lava	cola	month	triangle	five	blanket	bed		
molten metal	cloud	paper	France	pie	maths	subway		
pomp	music	fur	piano keyboard	pills	cow	wallet		
glue	wrist	tiger	clown	jam	milk	watch	sand	lake
chilli	pepper	stone	kitten	map	quaver	baboon	stick	
carrot	hitch	Paris	furnace	broach	rat	diamond	Spain	
paprika	French flag	guitar	goat	wallpaper paste	square			
bag	carrot	flipper	horizon	swimming	Brazil	deer		
brick	hot tarmac	hamster	antelope	balloon	conductor			
kangaroo	nice	radio	Cuba	underwear	honey	alphabet		
car	curry	sergeant's chevrons						

What strategies did you use to complete this task?

How did you find this exercise? Easy ☐ OK ☐ Quite difficult ☐ Very difficult ☐

EXERCISE 22

Count the 'THEs'

How difficult do you think you will find this exercise? Easy ☐ OK ☐ Quite difficult ☐ Very difficult ☐

Instruction

Read the following passage out loud. Everybody else has to count the number of times the word 'the' is mentioned. To make this exercise easier, people can follow the text on paper as it is being read.

UNPICKING THE LOCK

Beethoven's secret revealed in his hair

The life and work of Beethoven raise a number of intertwined questions. What made him so odd: clumsy; socially maladroit; ugly enough for a woman to whom he proposed to reject him for that alone; wildly irascible; increasingly in later life reclusive and paranoid? What caused him to lose his hearing before he was even 30? And – a question transcending all others – what was it that made him one of the two or three greatest composers in the history of music?

New evidence from the United States suggests that some or possibly all of these things had something to do with lead. He was ill from his youth with a number of wretched conditions, especially dysentry. In 1802 he wrote to his brothers lamenting his fate and saying the onset of deafness had brought him to the brink of despair and close to ending his life. He survived: but his problems grew worse. Now researchers in Chicago who have examined a lock of his hair believe he was suffering from lead poisoning. The concentrations they found in the hair were 100 times the level of lead which is common today.

The deaths of composers are often mysterious. Did Salieri murder Mozart? Did Tchaikovsky kill himself? There are plans to exhume Bellini, who may, some now think, have paid the ultimate price for taking a woman away from her previous lover. At least in Beethoven's case murder is not alleged – yet. Drinking water, food or utensils are listed as possible culprits.

We know how much the world would have lost had the composer's despair overwhelmed him in 1802. What we cannot tell is whether the music he wrote was shaped for better or worse by his malady.

What strategies did you use to complete this task?

How did you find this exercise? Easy ☐ OK ☐ Quite difficult ☐ Very difficult ☐

Count the 'OFs'

How difficult do you think you will find this exercise? Easy ☐ OK ☐ Quite difficult ☐ Very difficult ☐

Instruction

Read the following passage out loud. Everybody else has to count the number of times the word 'of' is mentioned. To make this exercise easier, people can follow the text on paper as it is being read.

An increase in the cost of vital home care services used by the elderly, infirmed and disabled has been condemned by care groups and pensioners. The cost of services such as meals on wheels, day centre provision and home helps is set to rise in April following a decision by the Berkshire social services committee meeting on Thursday 18 January.

Pensioners will also be hit by the level of Disability Living Allowance paid back to the council for domiciliary services rising from 20 per cent to 50 per cent.

It is estimated the higher charges will net the council an additional £590,000 – £50,000 of which has been earmarked for three new welfare benefit officers.

Jill Smith, who chairs Age Concern, said charges are spiraling 'out of control'. She said: 'All these higher charges will affect the most vulnerable sets of people in the community and it is just not on.'

Mrs Smith also feels that many elderly people are reluctant – or unable – to complain, making them an easy target for higher charges. She added: 'Pensioners often do not stand up for themselves, and I feel that these sorts of charges are spiraling out of control.'

The changes, recommended in an Audit Commission document, were described in a report to councilors as the 'fairest way possible' of increasing revenue.

The report said: 'Local authorities have to balance concerns about charging vulnerable users with the ever-increasing need to fund the service. Managers have to reconcile the need to generate income with the potential negative effects of charging, such as the anxiety charges can cause to users, and the cost of administering the charges.'

What strategies did you use to complete this task?

How did you find this exercise? Easy ☐ OK ☐ Quite difficult ☐ Very difficult ☐

Count the 'ANDs'

How difficult do you think you will find this exercise? Easy ☐ OK ☐ Quite difficult ☐ Very difficult ☐

Instruction

Read the following passage out loud. Everybody else has to count the number of times the word 'and' is mentioned. To make this exercise easier, people can follow the text on paper as it is being read.

BIRDS SET ALIGHT IN ART STUNT

Horrified shoppers and young children saw pigeons being set alight as part of an arts festival. They have branded the bizarre ritual by a Spanish artist as 'sick' and outraged officials of the Royal Society for the Protection of Birds fear some people will copy the stunt.

Controversial Jose Pallerno and his assistant used pigeons found dead on the streets for their act. But passers-by had no idea that was the case when they saw them blazing. Jose's act was part of the Manchester Biennial arts festival. When one angry shopper confronted him, he was told: 'I am burning my brothers.'

Jose said yesterday: 'I love pigeons very much and it's not nice to see them dying on the street, squashed by cars. I wanted to do something related to the area, so I chose to work with pigeons, which symbolise the North and the working classes.'

But Madeleine Pursley of the RSPB, said: 'We're horrified that anyone could justify this as an art form and hope that no one else would entertain doing anything like this.'

This is not the first time that Jose Pallerno has been in the news; two years ago, as part of the Barcelona Arts Festival, he produced a work that stunned and shocked art lovers everywhere. His piece, entitled Blood and Guts, consisted of two hundred and fifty metres of freshly slaughtered bulls' intestines, supported on six thousand matchsticks.

What strategies did you use to complete this task?

How did you find this exercise? Easy ☐ OK ☐ Quite difficult ☐ Very difficult ☐

Keeping in mind

How difficult do you think you will find this exercise? Easy ☐ OK ☐ Quite difficult ☐ Very difficult ☐

Instruction

This exercise is aimed at improving your ability to think of more than one thing at a time. Carry out the calculations below while following these three rules.

Rules

- When you see the symbol *, it means carry out the opposite calculation – the opposite sign – from the sum before. So if the calculation before had a plus (add) sign (+), then the * indicates minus (–) sign.
- When you see X in front of a calculation, it means stop working on this column immediately, do not carry out that calculation. Add up the total of the column, and move to the top of the next column and continue your calculations.
- When you see M in front of a calculation, it means miss out this calculation and go to the next one.

7 + 2 =	2 – 1 =	5 + 4 =	5 + 2 =
2 + 3 =	M 5 + 8 =	7 * 3 =	7 – 6 =
4 – 2 =	9 – 6 =	8 – 5 =	5 * 3 =
6 + 2 =	3 * 4 =	4 * 3 =	3 – 2 =
5 * 2 =	2 + 7 =	7 * 2 =	6 * 2 =
6 – 4 =	3 * 2 =	M 5 + 5 =	5 – 4 =
M 7 + 4 =	M 6 + 2 =	1 – 1 =	M 9 + 3 =
9 – 7 =	3 – 3 =	2 + 3 =	1 + 2 =
M 8 – 3 =	4 + 2 =	M 4 – 3 =	3 + 4 =
5 * 1 =	6 + 6=	5 + 5 =	5 – 3 =
4 + 5 =	X 7 + 4 =	6 – 3 =	2 + 3 =
3 + 4 =	2 + 2=	M 6 + 6 =	9 * 4 =
X 6 + 3 =	9 * 6 =	3 + 3 =	X 4 – 3 =
6 – 4 =	1 – 1 =	X 2 + 1 =	2 + 6 =
2 * 5 =	3 + 3 =	1 + 2 =	8 * 8 =
1 + 4 =	7 + 1 =	8 + 9 =	7 – 2 =
Total =	**Total =**	**Total =**	**Total =**

What strategies did you adopt to do this task?

How did you find this exercise? Easy ☐ OK ☐ Quite difficult ☐ Very difficult ☐

Dividing and switching attention

How difficult do you think you will find this exercise? Easy ☐ OK ☐ Quite difficult ☐ Very difficult ☐

Instructions

1 **Boys' and girls' names.** Go through the alphabet, and think of people's names beginning with each letter. However, alternate or switch between boys' and girls' names for each letter. This can be carried out in a group or individually, and can be presented on paper or verbally.

2 **Animals' and place-names.** Go through the alphabet, and alternately think of animal names and then place-names beginning with each letter. Again, this can be carried out individually, in a group, on paper or verbally. If it is too difficult, alter it by not having to follow the letters of the alphabet.

3 **Adding up the odd numbers.** Somebody reads out a list or row of numbers, quite slowly – one every second – and the group has to add up all the odd numbers. An easier version is just to keep a tally of how many odd numbers have been read out.

5 4 3 6 8 2 1 3 4 8 5 2 3 4 4 9 2 3 2 3 6 8 7 2 4 5 1 4 6 5 6
5 8 2 1 3 6 8 9 2 3 2 6 4 3 6 2 1 4 5 2 5 7 8 8 9 3 2 5 6 4 3
2 4 8 3 5 6 4 2 7 2 1 6 8 5 2 9 4 3 2 5 8 9 2 3 5 2 5 4 3 6 8
2 1 3 4 8 5 2 7 4 4 9 2 3 2 3 6 8 7 2 4 5 1 4 6 5 6 5 8 2 1 3

1 *Can you think of any situations in everyday life where you have to switch attention as you have done in this exercise?*
2 *What strategies did you use to carry out this task?*

How did you find this exercise? Easy ☐ OK ☐ Quite difficult ☐ Very difficult ☐

N-back exercise

How difficult do you think you will find this exercise? Easy ☐ OK ☐ Quite difficult ☐ Very difficult ☐

Instruction

This is a good exercise for 'sustained attention', and can be made as easy or difficult as you like by increasing or decreasing the number back from the responder.

1 **Warm up**. Go around the group: each person has to think up the name of an animal (or person's name, or place-name, or food) beginning with the next letter of the alphabet.
For example:

Person 1 'Aardvark'
Person 2 'Bear'
Person 3 'Cat'
Person 4 'Dog'

2 **One-back**. Go around the group in the same way, but this time each person has to name the previous person's animal, then one of their own.
For example:

Person 1 'Aardvark'
Person 2 'Aardvark, bear'
Person 3 'Bear, cat'
Person 4 'Cat, dog'

3 **Two-back**. Go around the group in the same way, but this time each person should say the previous person's animal but one, before their own. You have to focus on what the person two places away has said.
For example:

Person 1 'Aardvark'
Person 2 'Bear'
Person 3 'Aardvark, cat'
Person 4 'Bear, dog'

Ensure that a different person begins each round each time.

What strategies are effective for successfully completing this exercise?

How did you find this exercise? Easy ☐ OK ☐ Quite difficult ☐ Very difficult ☐

Have I got an attention problem?

How difficult do you think you will find this exercise? Easy ☐ OK ☐ Quite difficult ☐ Very difficult ☐

Instruction

1 Do you have any of the following problems? Which are the three most noticeable?

		Yes/No
1	Slower at processing information, so don't take in everything	
2	Easily distracted - drift off	
3	Can't filter out background noise	
4	Do not see things as clearly in my left visual field – visual neglect	
5	Difficulty doing two things at once	
6	Difficulty concentrating for long periods	
7	Difficulty switching attention	

2 Which of these strategies do you use for coping?

		Yes/No
1	Use external aids, such as alarms, cue cards, or voice mail	
2	Take frequent breaks	
3	Talk to myself during the task, saying things like 'stay focused'	
4	Tell other people that I've got a problem – enlist their help	
5	Work at my best time – when I'm not tired	
6	Practise a specific task that I'm not good at – gradually increasing the difficulty	
7	Rearrange my environment to exclude distractions and noise	

Give an example of a real-life occasion when you have deliberately used a coping strategy to improve your attention.

How did you find this exercise? Easy ☐ OK ☐ Quite difficult ☐ Very difficult ☐

Executive Skills

INFORMATION SHEETS

EXECUTIVE SKILLS EXERCISES

Executive skills questionnaire

Name ______________________________ Date ____________________

This questionnaire assesses your executive skills. Read each of the statements and mark the box that best describes your behaviour at present. It might be helpful to ask someone who knows you well to complete the questionnaire and fill in the independent scorer column.

Scoring Agree = 2 Partially agree = 1 Disagree = 0

Question	**Score**					
	Self-score			Independent scorer		
	Agree	Partially agree	Disagree	Agree	Partially agree	Disagree
1 I have difficulty planning and organising.						
2 I have difficulty doing more than one thing at a time.						
3 I have difficulty weighing up the pros and cons, deciding on what is important and making decisions.						
4 I sometimes misinterpret the actions of others and 'get the wrong end of the stick'.						
5 I am more impulsive, acting without thinking of the consequences.						
6 I often 'go off at tangents', or move too quickly from one idea to the other in conversation.						
7 I have difficulty summarising information, 'getting to the point', or 'seeing the wood from the trees'.						
8 I tend to hold firm, 'black and white' or rigid views.						
9 I have problems planning realistic goals, and working out the steps to achieve those goals.						
10 I sometimes have difficulty switching attention quickly in a fast-flowing conversation.						
TOTAL SCORE						

INTERPRETATION

Self-score

10–20: This suggests that your executive skills could be improved.

Discrepancy between self-score and independent score

5–20: This suggests that you may not be fully aware of your executive skills problems, or are denying them.

How relevant did you find this sheet? Very ☐ Slightly ☐ Not very ☐

Executive skills: what are they?

What are executive skills? Think of the skills that a typical good management executive requires. He needs to plan; organise; direct; control; set realistic goals; organise the steps to achieve those goals; initiate action programmes; monitor progress; and adjust those plans. He also needs to be aware of what is happening in sales, marketing and production, and to synthesise and analyse that information; make multiple decisions, and exercise good judgement. These are executive skills. However, it is not only executives who need these skills; we all use them a great deal in our everyday lives. They are vital to our ability to function independently at work, in the home, or when socialising.

The managing director or conductor. Executive skills can be thought of as the managing director or conductor of all other cognitive functions. The majority of cognitive functions are concerned with what we do; the executive skills relate to how we do it. Think of the executive skills as the conductor of an orchestra, and the cognitive skills as the various sections of the orchestra. If the conductor is not working properly then each part of the orchestra may play out of order, at the wrong volume, or at the wrong speed. In the same way, if the executive skills are not working well, then all other brain functions may be coordinated incorrectly on tasks – leading to significant problems in everyday life.

Located in the frontal lobes. These types of skills tend to be located in the frontal lobes of the brain (at the front, behind the forehead). This part of the brain is connected to all other brain areas, and 'communicates' with them with a rich interchange of information. The frontal area is often injured in a brain injury, particularly if there is an acceleration-deceleration injury when the brain is likely to grind into the front of the skull, and on to the bones above the eye sockets.

Hidden problems more noticeable in unstructured situations. Problems with executive skills tend to show themselves in unstructured situations. Therefore the problems are not easily observed in formal tests, which provide a structure. The problems may appear to be variable, since the complexity, novelty and amount of structure provided in any given task also varies with the situation. So, many people are not aware of difficulties in this area of function. Often people describe things as 'not being quite right', but are not able to describe the problems in more detail. Because of the nature of these problems, it is often very hard for the brain-injured person to recognise the difficulties in themselves.

Components of executive skills. Executive functions are divided into various skills. Here, we have broken them down for ease of recall, so that most of them begin with the letter 'S':

(i) *Stepping back:* The ability to step back and view a situation objectively, from a distance, rather than charging in impulsively without thinking.

Executive skills: what are they?

(ii) *Starting:* Self-initiation or starting an activity without help or prompting from anyone else.

(iii) *Sequencing and planning:* The ability to break down an overall goal into a number of discreet, achievable steps or sequences and then follow those steps. This is at the heart of the ability to plan and organise.

(iv) *Summarising:* The ability to see what is important – the main point – and what is a minor detail; then to gather together all the information and summarise it.

(v) *Staying online, or sustained attention:* The important skill of sustaining attention – not being distracted by irrelevancies; staying focused.

(vi) *Self-monitoring:* The ability to assess the appropriateness and effectiveness of what is done, and to be able to identify mistakes and careless errors.

(vii) *Shifting, switching and solving problems:* The ability to recognise a problem; work out an alternative solution, and then shift the pattern of responding to a new pattern. This involves switching attention.

(viii) *Stopping:* The ability to inhibit, or stop, expressing thoughts or behaviours that are inappropriate. We can all think or feel things, but sometimes we have to 'keep a lid' on them.

(ix) *Self-awareness:* The ability to have an accurate idea of our own strengths and weaknesses, and to be able to anticipate future difficulties.

Dysexecutive syndrome. This cluster of difficulties is sometimes known as the 'dysexecutive syndrome', or as a failure in the 'supervisory attention system' or 'frontal lobe syndrome'. People with these difficulties often present very well on casual acquaintance, and may convince people that they have well-formulated plans and goals, but they often have difficulty carrying them out.

1 Describe what you understand by the term 'executive skills'.
2 What do a 'managing director', a 'conductor' and the frontal lobes have in common?
3 When are problems with executive skills most likely to show themselves?
4 Name as many components of executive skills as you can. Nine are listed, all beginning with the letter 'S'.

How relevant did you find this sheet? Very ☐ Slightly ☐ Not very ☐

Ways of improving executive skills

Stepping back

- Take a step back – don't rush in. Think about it for a few moments.

Starting, or initiation

- Ask yourself the following questions and provide short clear answers:
  - (a) What is it I want to achieve?
  - (b) What do I need to do to move from my present situation to my goal?
  - (c) What options are available?
  - (d) What is the best option?
- Set yourself a specific goal.
- If you have a problem getting started, reward yourself for achieving specific tasks.

Sequencing and planning

- Make a list of the steps needed to achieve the task.
- Simplify the task – break it down into small steps, and write these down.
- Follow the steps in the correct order, perhaps ticking off each one as you have achieved it.

Summarising

- Try to identify the main points and the details – what is important and what is not important?
- Imagine you are above the information – try to get 'helicopter vision'.
- Talk to yourself by starting and finishing the sentence, 'The main idea is...'

Staying online, or sustained attention

- Remove distractions.
- Talk to yourself: at first, speak out loud; then whisper, and then talk silently to yourself, to remind yourself to stay focused.
- Use external cues, such as cue cards or bleeping watches.
- Work at your best time of day – not when you are tired.
- Take breaks.
- In the middle of tasks, check everything is going according to plan.

Self-monitoring

- Ask yourself the following questions, and provide short clear answers to them:
  - (a) How will I know that my plan has been successful?
  - (b) Have I achieved what I want to accomplish?
- Use checklists and always check your work.
- Get feedback from others. Ask them to be honest and direct.
- Video feedback is helpful.

Shifting or solving problems

- Look at, and recognise, errors and then do the task differently.
- Try to be flexible. Ask yourself, 'What are the other options?'
- Look at the problem from a different angle. Ask yourself how someone else might think.
- Allow longer to do the task.

Ways of improving executive skills

Stopping, or self-inhibition
- ➤ Ask for feedback from others – 'Tell me if I'm a bit over the top.'
- ➤ Question yourself, 'Have I overdone it?'
- ➤ Look out for how others are reacting.

Self-awareness
- ➤ Identify your strengths and weaknesses.
- ➤ Ask for feedback.
- ➤ Watch yourself on video.
- ➤ Predict how well you will do on a task, and then see how you do.
- ➤ Write a report after the task is done, identifying those things that you did well and the things that were not done so well.

1 Add any other ways of improving executive skills that you can think of under each individual section.

2 Which of these individual executive skills is your biggest problem?

3 What are the two most effective individual steps that you personally take to improve your executive skills?

➤

➤

How relevant did you find this sheet? Very ☐ Slightly ☐ Not very ☐

Some useful stategies for coping with executive problems

Recognise that you have a problem. Recognise that you probably have to think things through more deliberately, more consciously, whereas before executive thinking might have been more automatic.

Step back – survey – pause. Take a step back, and survey the situation. Try not to jump in 'head first'.

Problem solve by asking yourself key questions. What am I trying to achieve? What are the options or solutions? Weigh up the pros and cons of each possible solution. Decide on the best solution. Plan the steps involved to reach that solution or goal.

Make a plan or a list – write it down. Making a list can help to sort out what it is you need to do. It can then also help you to make sure you get everything done. Tick off each item on the list.

Check and double check. Monitoring what you are doing. Ask yourself, 'Am I still on track? Is my solution working? Have I made any careless errors?' Adjust your plan if necessary. Stand back and make an overall evaluation.

Talk to yourself. Talking yourself through a set of instructions or a problem, either in your head, or even better out loud, can help to make things clearer.

Remove distraction. This may mean going off into a quiet room, shutting the door, turning off the TV, or putting the answering machine on.

Take frequent breaks. Do not work over one hour without a break.

Use a wall calendar. Put all appointments on a wall calendar.

Use a large white board. Helpful for mapping out problems, or making plans, and allows you the option of literally stepping back to look at a problem.

Carry a diary or small notebook. Useful for jotting down ideas, taking messages, or writing lists.

Be tidier and more organised. One person said that he could cope with a disorganised desk before his brain injury, because he knew where everything was, but since his accident everything had to be very organised and neat, otherwise he could not cope.

Ask for advice and feedback. Get someone you trust to give you feedback. It helps to have another point of view.

Be assertive – delegate and 'say no'. If you recognise that you can no longer do the task, delegate it to someone else whom you trust or say 'no'.

Some useful stategies for coping with executive problems

Steps Involved in Problem Solving in Executive Tasks

Step back and identify the main problem.
(What am I trying to achieve?)

⇓

What are the options or possible solutions?

⇓

What is the best option?
(Weigh up the pros and cons of each.)

⇓

Plan out the steps involved to reach the solution.
(Think about timing and strategies.)

⇓

Carry out the plan.

⇓

Monitor progress and adjust plan accordingly.
(Ask yourself 'Am I still on track? Is it working?')

⇓

Evaluate.
(Was it a success – what were the positives and negatives?)

How relevant did you find this sheet? Very ☐ Slightly ☐ Not very ☐

Executive skills quiz

1 How bad do you think your executive skills are, compared with before your injury?

The same ☐ Slightly worse ☐ Much worse ☐

2 From the list below, mark those skills that are executive skills with a tick:

Planning and organising	Doing two things at the same time
Remembering your childhood	Seeing both sides of an argument
Speaking a foreign language	Making decisions
Noticing when you make a mistake	Working towards set goals
Good eyesight	The ability to summarise information

3 Which part of the brain do executive skills tend to be associated with?

____

____

4 What do the managing director of a company, a military general, and the conductor of an orchestra have in common, with the frontal lobes of the brain?

____

____

5 Identify three practical strategies you could use to help with, or compensate for, your executive skills difficulties.

____

____

6 Which of the following jobs would be most suited to, and least suited to, a person with significant executive skills deficits? Rank in order and then discuss.

	Working on the till in a busy McDonalds restaurant
	Working in a garden centre looking after the bedding plants
	Managing a large furniture removals company

How relevant did you find this sheet? Very ☐ Slightly ☐ Not very ☐

EXERCISE 1

The main idea – birthday letter

How difficult do you think you will find this exercise? Easy ☐ OK ☐ Quite difficult ☐ Very difficult ☐

Instruction

The aim of this exercise is to help you summarise, or 'see the wood for the trees'. Read the letter carefully, and then answer the questions that follow.

> Dear Jane
>
> Thank you for helping me plan Larry's 60th birthday party. I have been thinking about a number of possible dates, and would like to get your opinion on them. On 5 August, possibly the six of us could surprise him with tickets for a show in London – *South Pacific* is back, and he loves old musicals. He is also free on 12 August. Rachael suggested we keep it simple, and just get the family together for a meal and leave it at that. She and Harry are free on either the 5th or the 12th. Margaret and Ralph rang last week and told me they would like to be involved, especially if we have a party – they are free on the 5th and the 10th, but not the 12th. What about a barbecue if the weather is fine? What do you think? Please call me next week, preferably early evening and we can come up with a plan. Thanks.
>
> Yours, Helen

1 Choose one of the following options which best describes what the letter is about:

(a) How old Larry is
(b) Who Larry's relatives are
(c) When Larry's birthday should be celebrated
(d) Who should come to the birthday celebration

2 Which of the following sentences reflect the main idea of the letter and which describe details? Place an 'M' in front of the one main idea, and a 'D' in front of the sentences that describe details:

_____ Larry's 60th birthday is rapidly approaching
_____ Helen would like a barbecue if the weather is fine
_____ Margaret and Ralph would like to be involved and come to the party
_____ Helen wants Jane's opinion regarding plans for Larry's birthday

3 Which of the following statements captures the purpose of the letter?

(a) To express annoyance over the problems involved with organising the party
(b) To request input regarding various dates for Larry's party
(c) To persuade Jane to come to a barbecue
(d) To invite everybody along to a family meal

4 Describe one minor detail of the letter.

____

5 Summarise the letter in a maximum of six words for a telegram or text message.

____

How relevant did you find this sheet? Very ☐ Slightly ☐ Not very ☐

The main idea – holiday letter

How difficult do you think you will find this exercise? Easy ☐ OK ☐ Quite difficult ☐ Very difficult ☐

Instruction

The aim of this exercise is to help you summarise, or 'see the wood for the trees'. Read the letter carefully, and then answer the questions that follow.

> Dear Customer
>
> I am pleased to be able to send you our annual newsletter and magazine. It has been a very good year with a record number of satisfied holidaymakers. Enclosed is next year's listings of our SUN LINE cruise schedule. As you will see, we have a new cruise around the Caribbean. We also have a special incentive, which is bound to spark your interest. If you register for a SUN LINE cruise before September, we will provide four days' stay at a resort hotel of your choice – either before or after your trip. The offer is limited, so if you are interested please respond quickly. Other features of our new season include expanded celebrity-filled shows, on-board saunas and health suites and refurbished casinos on the sun decks of all our ships. So sign up for a SUN LINE tour now. We would like to take you on a holiday of a lifetime.
>
> SUN LINE TOURS

1 Choose one of the following options which best describes what the letter is about:

(a) Where the cruises are going
(b) Who is eligible for the cruise
(c) The ships have been refurbished
(d) What the cruise line is offering

2 Which of the following sentences reflect the main idea of the letter and which describe details? Place an 'M' in front of the main idea, and a 'D' in front of the sentences that describe details.

_____ SUN LINE is offering a free four-day stay in a hotel if you book a cruise now
_____ The cruise line is trying to entice customers to make reservations
_____ It's been a good year for SUN LINE and they want to publicise it
_____ The refurbished casino is on the sun deck

3 Which one of the following statements captures the purpose of the letter?

(a) Persuade travellers to visit Ibiza
(b) Discourage gambling on the ship
(c) Inform the reader of what value for money a SUN LINE cruise is
(d) Encourage customers to take a trip on a SUN LINE cruise

4 Describe one minor detail of the letter.

____

____

5 Summarise the letter in a maximum of eight words for a telegram or text message:

____

____

How relevant did you find this sheet? Very ☐ Slightly ☐ Not very ☐

The main idea – letter home

How difficult do you think you will find this exercise? Easy ☐ OK ☐ Quite difficult ☐ Very difficult ☐

Instruction

The aim of this exercise is to help you summarise, or 'see the wood for the trees'. Read the letter carefully, and then answer the questions that follow.

Dear Mum and Dad

The plane got in at 12.40 on Tuesday, almost an hour late because there was a security alert at the airport. It must have been a bomb scare, because I'd never seen so many police – no bomb though. The heat and humidity hit us like a wall when we stepped off the plane, but thankfully our hotel room is air-conditioned. Kathy sends her love, as does cousin Frank whom we met yesterday for the first time. He flew in from New Zealand on Saturday – so he knows his way around. The streets are crowded with rickshaws, lorries, cars and sacred cows. Anyway, we are safe and well and enjoying the trip so far. Oh by the way, if you've got time, could you let Mike know that I'll be away for three weeks – although I'm sure Jack will tell him, so don't bother unless you see him. Must go now as the Post Office is just about to shut – what a splendid building it is – huge high glass ceiling – very inefficient counter staff though. We will write later in more detail – possibly next week.

Lots of love, Brian.

1 Write one sentence that reflects the main point or purpose of the letter.

____

____

2 Write a sentence that describes one important detail of the letter.

____

____

3 Write a sentence that describes one trivial, unimportant detail.

____

____

4 How many people are mentioned in the paragraph, and how are they related?

____

____

How relevant did you find this sheet? Very ☐ Slightly ☐ Not very ☐

The main idea – text message

How difficult do you think you will find this exercise? Easy ☐ OK ☐ Quite difficult ☐ Very difficult ☐

Instruction

You are desperate to get an important message through to your girlfriend, and have written her an email, which has not got through. Your only option is to text her a message on to her mobile phone. You therefore need to summarise your email letter and reduce it to just SEVEN key words.

Dear Sarah

I am so sorry about what happened on Friday night – I was completely in the wrong and should not have lost my temper and shouted at you in that way. Very sorry about knocking the flowers over as well and kicking the bedroom door. But you know my family – we are all just hot heads – it must be the Italian blood, or maybe it is all down to my relationship with my father. I am trying to control it. I'll try to get some therapy as you suggested. I know I can be difficult, but I would hate this to ruin our relationship. We need to talk. Will you meet me in the pub tonight after work at 6.30? Please, please be there. You know the one – I can't think of its name, but it's the one we always go to. I need to see you tonight because I've got to go away for a couple of weeks, probably to the States, on business. Please be there, Sarah. I don't want to go away without sorting this out. I will be there from 6 o'clock onward and will wait all night if necessary.

I love you.

Antonio

Text message (7 words only):

What strategies did you use to summarise this letter?

How relevant did you find this sheet? Very ☐ Slightly ☐ Not very ☐

EXERCISE 5

Classified ad

How difficult do you think you will find this exercise? Easy ☐ OK ☐ Quite difficult ☐ Very difficult ☐

Instruction

Design a classified advertisement using the following information:

You have a child's cabin bed that you wish to sell, as your son has grown out of it. You have owned the bed for five years, from new, and it has been well taken care of. However, there is a stain on the mattress, some writing in felt pen on the headboard, and one of the steps of the ladder is missing. It is made of pine, has an upper bunk, and below, a built-in desk with three drawers and a small built-in wardrobe. There is also a swivel office chair to go with the desk. The bed can be taken apart and easily reassembled using bolts and a special allen key. It is 200 centimetres long, 90 centimetres wide and 140 centimetres high. You need £80 for it, so that you can buy a new camera. The cost of the advert is £1 a line, and there are 6 words to the line. You only want to spend £3 on the advert.

Design your classified advertisement here, giving all the relevant information for a quick sale.

What strategies did you use to complete this task?

How did you find this exercise? Easy ☐ OK ☐ Quite difficult ☐ Very difficult ☐

EXERCISE 6

Two questions at a time

How difficult do you think you will find this exercise? Easy ☐ OK ☐ Quite difficult ☐ Very difficult ☐

Instruction

One person in the group – the quizmaster – asks a simple general knowledge question to each person in the group in turn. The catch is that when a question is asked, the person being asked must give the answer to the question given to the person *before* them. The aim of the exercise is to answer the questions quickly and keep concentration going for as long as possible.

Example: To person A: What is the capital of England?
To person B: What is the colour of snow?
Person B replies: London.

Note: The person who gets the first question will not be able to give an answer first time around. After a while, try making it harder by using a two question delay before the answer is given.

Examples of questions

Name an animal you would find in a zoo.	What is a rectangle?
Who is the British Prime Minister?	Name one famous tennis player.
Where is Paris?	What day is it today?
How many legs does a donkey have?	How many items in a score?
Name two vegetables.	What colour is a red cabbage?
What do you call a baby cow?	Name two kinds of alcoholic drink.
What is the capital of Australia?	What is your favorite coloured shirt?
What is a hammer for?	Who is the US President?
What is a small boat called?	How many in a dozen?
What day comes after Monday?	What colour is an orange?
What's another name for Father Christmas?	How many legs does a centipede have?
Where is Alaska?	How many legs does a spider have?
How many inches in a foot?	Where do you keep your money?
What is usually the colour of the sky?	Who was the previous Prime Minister?
What colour is grass?	What do you call the place where you live?

Write down and then discuss what strategies you use to selectively attend to the previous question.

How did you find this exercise? Easy ☐ OK ☐ Quite difficult ☐ Very difficult ☐

Moral dilemmas

How difficult do you think you will find this exercise? Easy ☐ OK ☐ Quite difficult ☐ Very difficult ☐

Instruction

In the following exercise, read the outline of the dilemma; then try to work out which factors or issues are most important to consider. Objectively list what might be important.

Robert's dilemma: Take the money and run?

Robert is a 53-year-old single social worker who lives on his own in a detached house with a large garden in a quiet suburban residential close. He has been happy in his house for the last 10 years, and gets on well with the other eight neighbours. A group of property developers have asked all the residents whether they would be willing to sell the bottom end of their gardens for a considerable sum of money – all have agreed. However, the developers have approached Robert independently and offered him £150,000 plus the value of his house if he will sell them the house and allow them to knock it down to build the approach road for this development. If the neighbours stick together, they can negotiate collectively with different developers, but if Robert sells his house unilaterally to one developer, that developer will then own the key piece of property, meaning that the neighbours would be in a weaker bargaining position if other developers came along. Robert's dilemma is whether to take the money or to stick with his neighbours.

What are the most important factors that Robert needs to consider and weigh up?

➤

➤

➤

➤

➤

How did you find this exercise? Easy ☐ OK ☐ Quite difficult ☐ Very difficult ☐

Thinking past the obvious

How difficult do you think you will find this exercise? Easy ☐ OK ☐ Quite difficult ☐ Very difficult ☐

Instruction

Think of four possible reasons for each of the following unusual situations – be as creative as possible:

A group of people wearing hats.

➤
➤
➤
➤

A crowd of people looking up at a building.

➤
➤
➤
➤

A group of seven-year-olds with jam jars.

➤
➤
➤
➤

A person with 40 punnets of strawberries in a supermarket trolley.

➤
➤
➤
➤

A woman with an empty pram.

➤
➤
➤
➤

Think of a bizarre situation of your own, and create four possible explanations.

How did you find this exercise? Easy ☐ OK ☐ Quite difficult ☐ Very difficult ☐

Theme park

How difficult do you think you will find this exercise? Easy ☐ OK ☐ Quite difficult ☐ Very difficult ☐

Instruction

Carefully plan a route around the theme park by marking the map, but keep to the following rules:

1. You cannot walk along the same path twice.
2. You must always keep to the paths.
3. You must visit the following areas: Snake House, Big Wheel, Runaway Train, Roller Coaster, Corkscrew Ride and Dolphin Show (2.30–3.15pm).
4. You start the day at 10.00am and have arranged to meet a friend for lunch at the café at 1.30pm. You have to leave at 3.30pm.
5. You would like to visit the gift shop last.

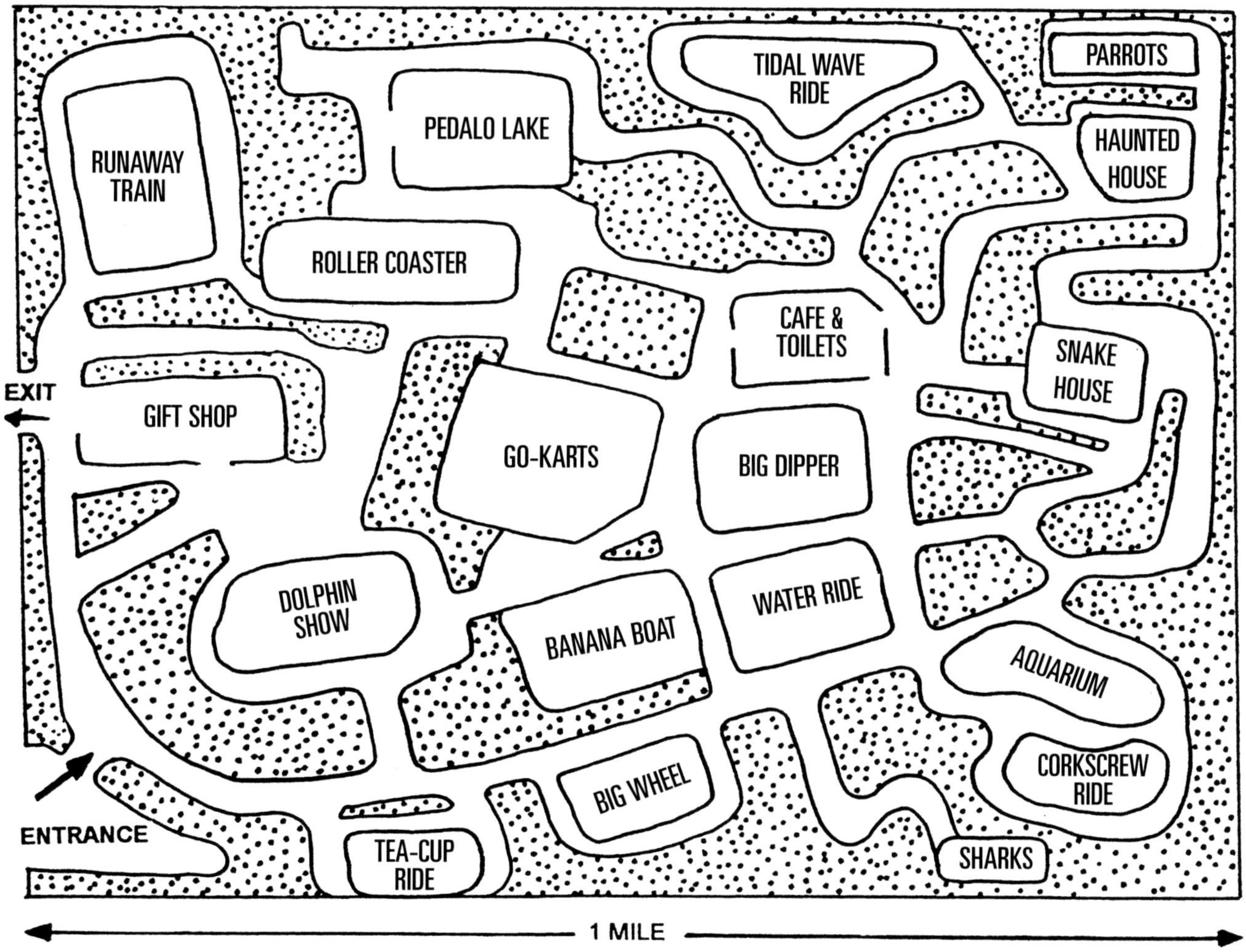

What strategies did you use to complete the task?

How did you find this exercise? Easy ☐ OK ☐ Quite difficult ☐ Very difficult ☐

EXERCISE 10

Woodley carnival

How difficult do you think you will find this exercise? Easy ☐ OK ☐ Quite difficult ☐ Very difficult ☐

Instruction

Imagine that you want to take photographs of the Woodley carnival procession, and need to plan a route to get the best positions for good photos. You have a bicycle and want to plan a route to zigzag across the map, so that you keep in front of the procession. The procession starts at Comet Way and finishes at the Carnival ground. Mark out your route on the map below, as you would on a maze, identifying seven positions to take photos, excluding position one, which is your starting and finishing point. You must keep to the following rules:

- The seven positions must be equally spread over the route.
- The thick black line on the map represents barriers along the pavement and cannot be crossed – it is also not easy to take good photos from behind the barrier.
- You can cross over the carnival route, but you must cross over the road directly.
- You cannot cycle down the carnival route.
- Finish where you started at Position 1.

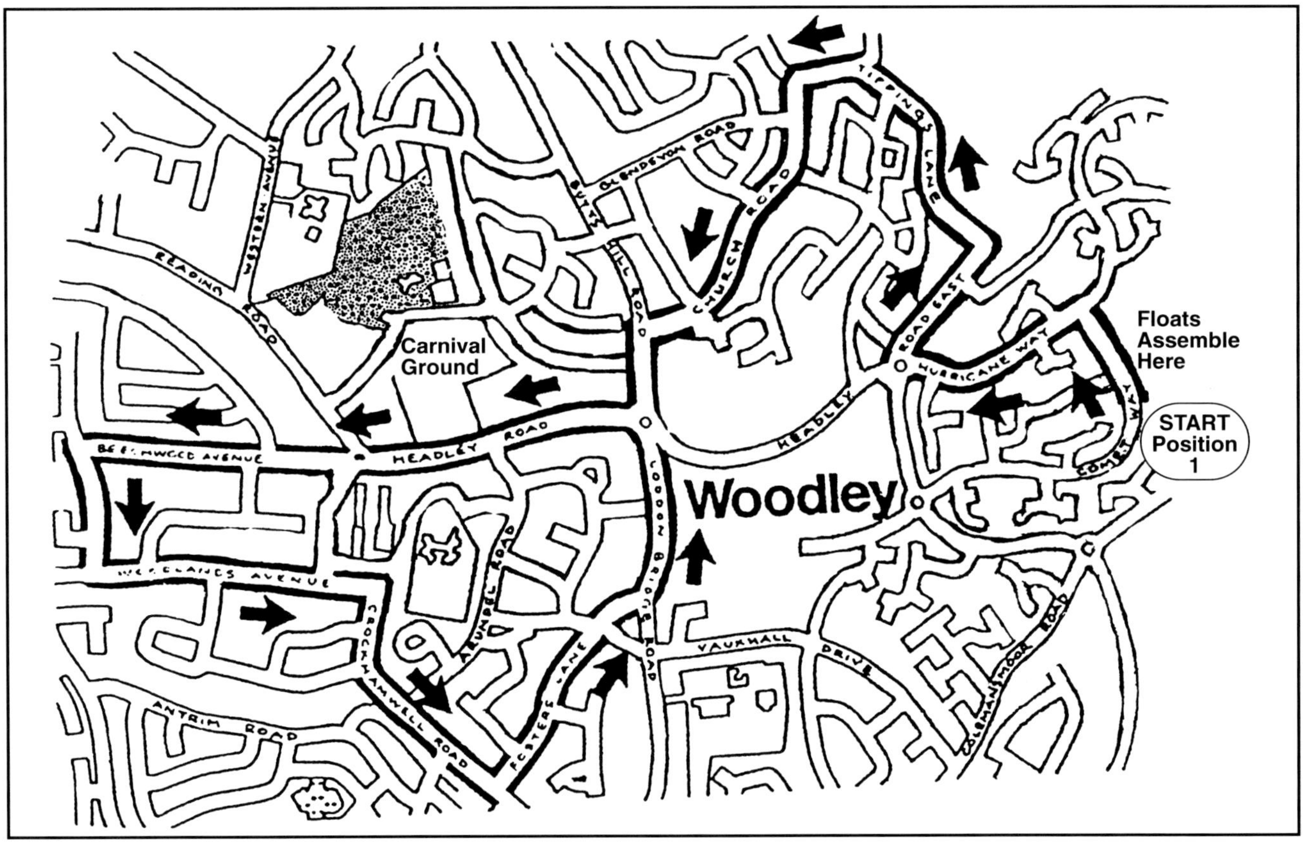

What strategy did you use to plan your route?

How did you find this exercise? Easy ☐ OK ☐ Quite difficult ☐ Very difficult ☐

Plan a day at the Dome

How difficult do you think you will find this exercise? Easy ☐ OK ☐ Quite difficult ☐ Very difficult ☐

Instruction

You and your family are going to the Leisure Dome. Plan your day using the map and the timetable, taking into account all the requirements for the day.

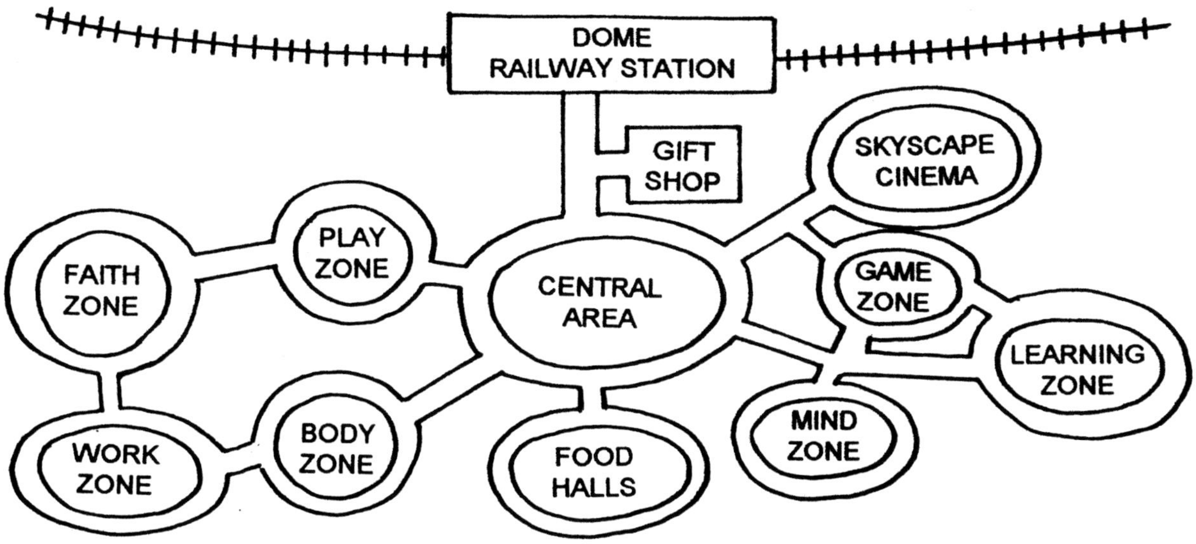

- Arrive at Dome station at 10.00am
- Need to be home by 7.30pm. Journey takes 2½ hours. Trains leave the station to go home at 2.00pm, 3.00pm, 3.30pm, 4.00pm, 4.45pm, 5.15pm, and 5.45pm.
- You want to see the show in the central area. Performances are at either 12.00 noon or 3.15pm. They run for 45 minutes.
- You want to see the special 30-minute Blackadder film, which is on at the Skyscape cinema at 11.45am, 12.45pm, 3.30pm and 4.30pm.
- You want to buy some souvenirs from the gift shop.
- You have arranged to meet some friends, Heather and Mark, for lunch in the Food Halls at one o'clock.
- You want to visit the following zones: Play Zone, Game Zone, Body Zone, Work Zone, Mind Zone.
- Allow approximately 30 minutes for each zone.
- Allow 5–10 minutes to walk between any two points on the map.

TIMETABLE
10.00am
11.00
12.00
1.00pm
2.00
3.00
4.00
5.00
6.00
7.00
8.00
9.00

How did you find this exercise? Easy ☐ OK ☐ Quite difficult ☐ Very difficult ☐

EXERCISE 12

Answer the question

How difficult do you think you will find this exercise? Easy ☐ OK ☐ Quite difficult ☐ Very difficult ☐

Instruction

Read ALL the questions before starting the exercise. Try to finish the exercise as quickly as possible.

1 What does $2 \times 2 \times 3$ equal?

2 Name two capital cities in Europe.

3 What colour do you get when you mix blue and yellow?

4 Write your name at the top of the paper.

5 Who do you think is the most powerful person in the world?

6 What is your favourite film?

7 What does $(3 \times 3) + (5 \times 2)$ equal

8 What is the third letter of the alphabet?

9 How many sides does a square have?

10 Now that you have read all the questions, go back and answer the first two questions only. Once you have answered the first two questions you have finished. You do not need to answer any other question.

This exercise is relevant to the problems of brain injury because it demonstrates how impulsive we can all be, jumping in head first without carefully weighing up what is required. This trait is particularly pronounced after a head injury. Think of a situation where you have been impulsive and write it down.

How did you find this exercise? Easy ☐ OK ☐ Quite difficult ☐ Very difficult ☐

One-minute presentation

How difficult do you think you will find this exercise? Easy ☐ OK ☐ Quite difficult ☐ Very difficult ☐

Instruction

Interview somebody in the group, or someone you know, finding out as much as you can about them. Allow yourself five minutes to do this. Your task is to give a one-minute presentation about the person that you have just interviewed. However, in the presentation you have to mention the following: 1) a job; 2) a number; 3) a wish; 4) a problem. To be successful, you must talk for one full minute, mention all four items, and provide relevant interesting information about the person. While others are giving their presentations, check whether they mention all four points.

Notes

Notes for presentation

Comments on others' presentations

How did you find this exercise? Easy ☐ OK ☐ Quite difficult ☐ Very difficult ☐

What are the emotions?

How difficult do you think you will find this exercise? Easy ☐ OK ☐ Quite difficult ☐ Very difficult ☐

Instruction

Look at the faces below, and on the line under each face write in which of the following moods fits most appropriately. There are 12 faces and 12 moods.

hostile	sorrow, tearful	very angry	sad
indifferent	sheepishly glad	worried	happy
disgusted	sceptical	run-down, tired	shocked

1

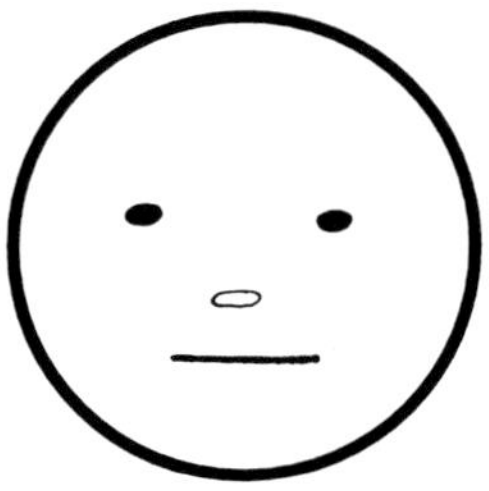

2

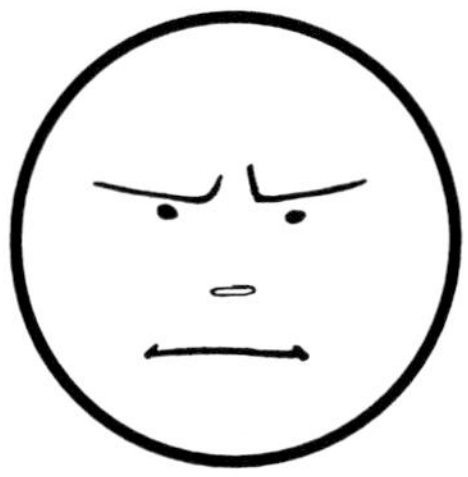

3

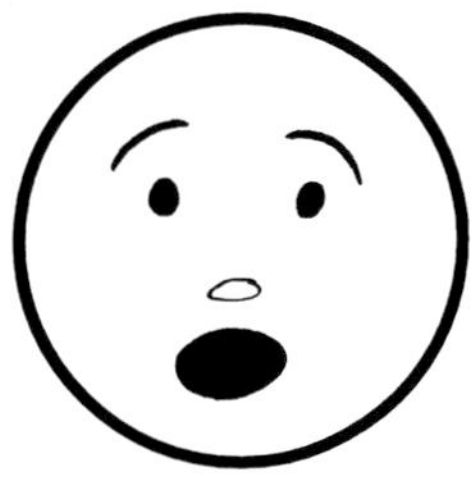

4

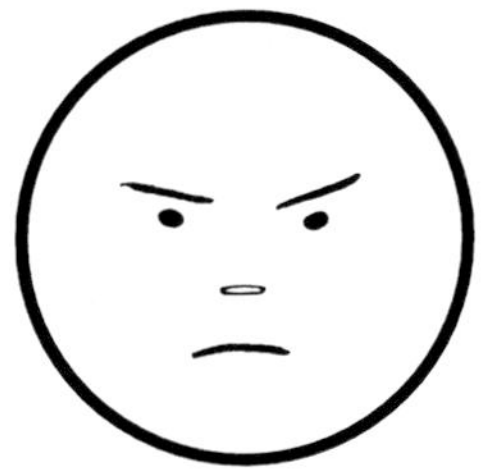

5

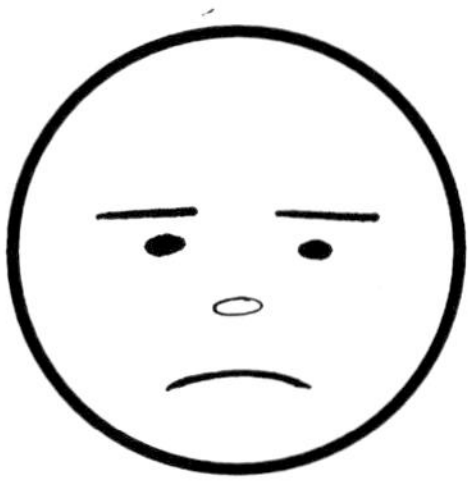

6

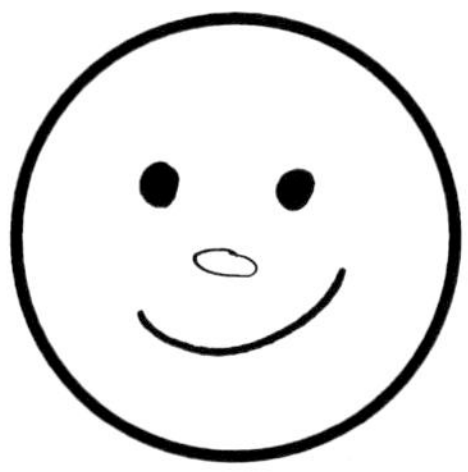

7

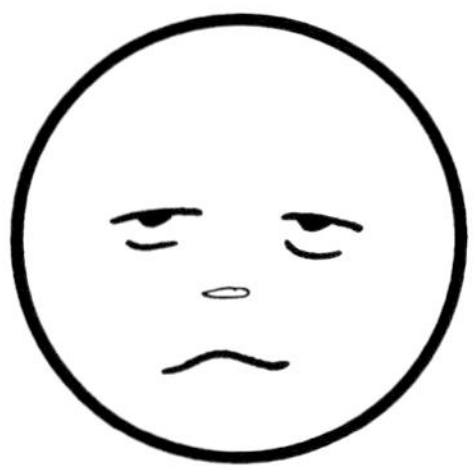

8

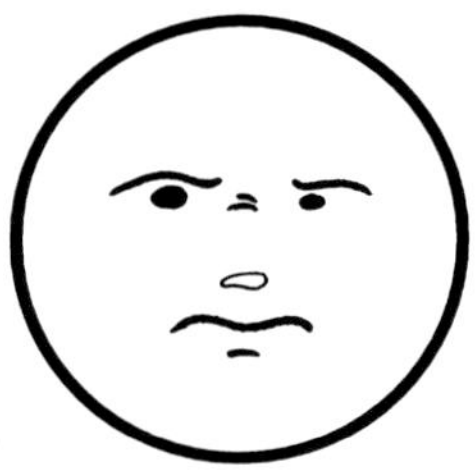

9

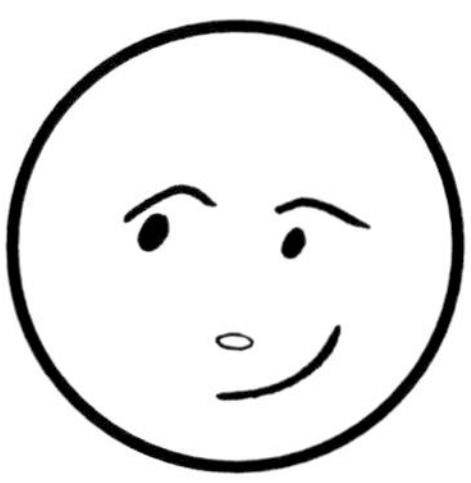

10

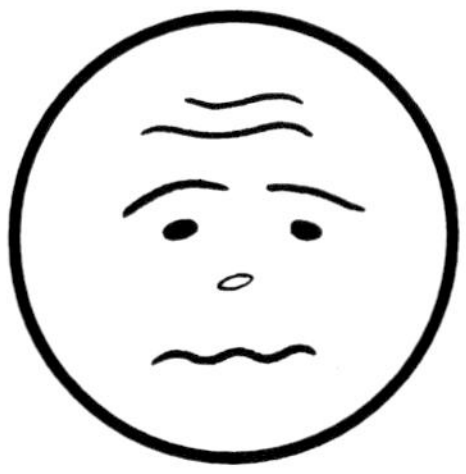

11

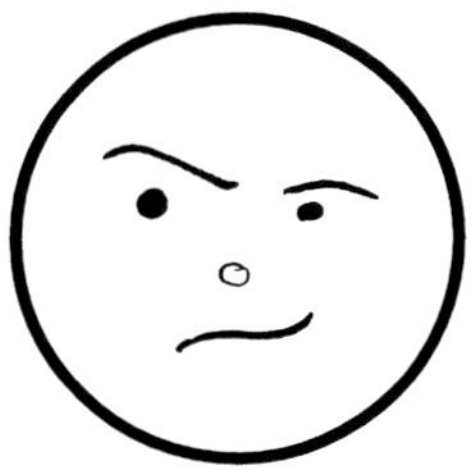

12

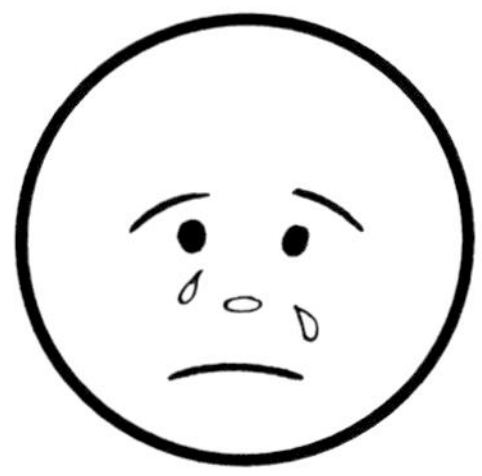

How did you find this exercise? Easy ☐ OK ☐ Quite difficult ☐ Very difficult ☐

Five activities task

How difficult do you think you will find this exercise? Easy ☐ OK ☐ Quite difficult ☐ Very difficult ☐

This is an executive skills task that involves multitasking and planning. The therapist reads through the instructions, identifies the equipment and the tasks, and keeps time.

Instruction

Follow the rules below to complete the task:

➤ You have 15 minutes to finish.
➤ There are five separate tasks.
➤ You have to completely finish at least one of the tasks.
➤ You have to complete the first two items of each task.

Equipment

➤ You will need a copy of the Yellow Pages (deliberately have fewer copies than there are people in the group).
➤ You will need a number of copies of the television listings (again, have fewer copies than the number of people in the group).

Tasks

1 Yellow Pages
2 Arithmetic
3 Television listings
4 Crosswords
5 Degraded letters (perceptual task)

Task 1: Yellow Pages

1 The wind has damaged your TV aerial. Identify the name and number of one firm who might help.

____

2 You want to go to the cinema. Find the numbers of two local cinemas.

____

3 You have a leaky roof. Find the name of a firm that offers 24-hour emergency cover.

____

4 You want to contact a solicitor who specialises in personal injury and will offer a free consultation. Find a name and telephone number.

____

5 You have some old cine-film, which you would like to transfer onto video. Find the name and telephone number of a company who could help.

____

Five activities task

Task 2: Arithmetic

1 36 + 28 =

2 7 + 11 =

3 267 – 86 =

4 741 – 125 =

5 347 – 21 =

6 25 x 5 =

7 19 x 12 =

8 8 x 24 =

Task 3: Television Listings

1 Which channel would you need to tune in to, so that you can watch live horse racing in the afternoon?

____

2 On which channel is there news at 1 o'clock lunchtime?

____

3 Your friend who is interested in Greek Philosophers has asked you to video a programme that is on in the mid-evening, but you have forgotten what it is called. Which programme is it most likely to be, and what channel is it on?

____

4 Your 12-year-old daughter wants to watch a pop chart programme. What time and channel is it on?

____

5 Your grandmother is coming to stay at 12.15pm, and she loves watching old black and white Hollywood films in the afternoon. Can you pick out a suitable film and identify the time and channel?

____

6 On which channel and at what time is there a mid-evening film? What is it about?

____

Five activities task

THURSDAY

Channel 1

6.00 Breakfast. (C) **9.00** Kilroy; (C) (S) BBC News; Weather. **10.00** City Hospital; (C) (S) BBC News; Weather. **11.00** Big Strong Boys. (C) (S) **11.30** Bargain Hunt; (C) (S) BBC News; Weather. **12.00** Wipeout. (R) (C) **12.30** Call My Bluff. With Eve Pollard. (C) (S) **1.00** BBC News; (C) Weather. **1.30** Regional News; Weather. **1.45** Neighbours. (C) (S) **2.10** Doctors. (C) (S) **2.40** Diagnosis Murder. (R) (C) (S) **3.25** CBeedbies: Tweenies Songtime. (C) (S) **3.26** Tweenies. (C) (S) **3.45** CBBC: Rugrats (R) (C) (S) **4.10** The Cramp Twins. (R) (C) (S) **4.25** The Story of Tracy Beaker. (C) (S) **4.35** The Mummy. Animation. (R) (C) (S)

5.00 Grange Hill. Tom keeps a secret, Ian acts strangely and Vikki finds herself sorely tempted. (C) (S)

5.25 Newsround. (C) (S)

5.35 Neighbours. (R) (C) (S)

6.00 BBC News. (C)

6.30 South Today; Weather.

7.00 Kabul Zoo Rescue. Jamie Darling travels to Afghanistan with the World Society for the Protection of Animals on a mission to improve conditions for creatures in Kabul Zoo and around the city. (C)

7.30 EastEnders. Pauline confronts Lisa about her secret meetings with Phil, Jamie tells Sonia he doesn't want children and Natalie realises Barry deliberately lied to Nathan about her birthday. (C) (S)

8.00 DIY SOS. Nick Knowles and the team travel to Stockton and create a calm living room to restore harmony to a couple torn apart by DIY. Plus, Lowri Turner presents more pleas for help. (C) (S)

8.30 This is Your Life. Michael Aspel pays tribute to another of the nation's stars or heroes. (C) (S)

9.00 Clocking Off. Gary thinks he's met the woman of his dreams, until she turns out to be a prostitute hired to steal his sizeable inheritance. (C)

10.00 BBC News at Ten O'Clock. (C)

10.25 Regional News; Weather.

10.35 Question Time. David Dimbleby chairs the topical political debate, as a panel of guests face questions from the audience. (C) (S)

11.35 Living Dangerously. (C) (S)

Channel 2

7.00 CBBC: Oscar's Orchestra. (R) (C) (S) **7.20** Arthur. (R) (C) **7.50** Blue Peter. (R) (C) (S) **8.15** CBeebies: Dr. Otter. (C) **8.25** Poddington Peas. (R) (C) **8.35** Postman Pat. (R) (C) **8.50** Pingu. (R) **9.00** Teletubbies. (R) (C) (S) **9.50** Playdays. (R) (C) (S) **10.10** Tweenies. (R) (C) (S) **10.50** Schools. **12.30** Working Lunch. **1.00** CBeebies: Dr. Otter. (R) (C) **1.10 FILM:** Beautiful But Dangerous (1952). Comedy, starring Jean Simmons. (C) (b/w) **2.35** Home Front Tricks. (C) **2.40** Westminster. (C) **3.20** BBC News; Regional News and Weather. (C) **3.30** Esther. (C) (S) **4.30** Ready Steady Cook. (C)

5.15 The Weakest Link. (C)

6.00 The Simpsons. (R) (C)

6.20 The Fresh Prince of Bel-Air. (R) (C)

6.45 Buffy the Vampire Slayer. Last in series. (C)

7.30 Southern Eye. The daughter of the Chief Constable of Sussex tells her story. (C)

8.00 Lifting the Bonnet. Sangita Myska and the team go undercover to reveal the growing problem of falsified motor documentation. (C) (S)

8.30 Wrong Car, Right Car. A Bristol schoolteacher trades in his unreliable Fiat Panda. (C) (S)

9.00 Horizon. The discovery of an ancient text written by Greek philosopher Archimedes. (C) (S)

9.55 Trouble at the Top. Nightspot owner Piers Adam plans an ambitious project which he hopes will change the face of clubbing in the UK forever. (C) (S)

10.30 Newsnight. (C)

11.20 Rugby Special. Jonathan Davies and Keith Wood present a special edition.

Channel 3

5.30 ITV Morning News. **6.00** GMTV. **9.25** Trisha. (T) (S) **10.30** This Morning. (T) **12.00** Family Fortunes. (R) (T) (S) **12.30** ITV Lunchtime News. (T) **1.05** Lunchtime Live on Meridian. (S) **1.40** Crossroads. (R) (T) (S) **2.10** Holidays from Hell 2. (R) (T) (S) **3.10** ITV News Headlines. (T) **3.15** Meridian News; Weather. (T) (S) **3.20** CITV: Dog and Duck. (T) (S) **3.30** Kipper (R) (T) (S) **3.40** Little Ghosts. (T) **3.50** Digimon. (R) (T) (S) **4.15** How 2. (R) (T) (S) **4.35** My Parents Are Aliens. (R) (T)

5.05 Night and Day. (T) (S)

5.30 Crossroads. Oona and Dave face a tough future. (T) (S)

6.00 Meridian Tonight; Weather. (T)

6.30 ITV Evening News; Weather. (T)

7.00 Emmerdale. The rivalry between Diane and Viv hots up, especially when Bob takes on more work at the Woolpack. (T) (S)

7.30 Tonight with Trevor McDonald. Topical issues. (T)

8.00 The Bill. Carver looks into a series of burglaries carried out while the victims were on holiday, and Singh is assigned to investigate an attack for which he was responsible. Drama, with Mark Wingett. (T)

9.00 Bad Girls. As an ecstatic Di announces her enagement to Barry, Shaz and Barbara go to great lengths to stop her from making the biggest mistake of her life, knowing just what a rat her intended really is. (T) (S)

10.00 ITV News at Ten; Weather. (T)

10.30 Baddiel and Skinner Unplanned. New series. Improvised repartee, with the duo holding forth on subjects suggested by the audience and rounding off each show with a rendition of a popular song. (T)

11.00 Night and Day. (T) (S)

CARLTON: 1.09 Carlton City Survival Guide. **1.10** London Today. **1.39** Carlton City Survival Guide. **3.08** Carlton City Survival Guide. **3.15** London Today. **3.19** Carlton City Survival Guide. Advice and information. **6.00** London Tonight. **11.58** Carlton Weather. **11.59** Carlton City Survival Guide. **12.00** Veronica's Closet. (S)

Channel 4

6.00 Grabbit the Rabbit. (R) (T) **6.10** The Hoobs. (R) (T) **6.35** The Hoobs. (R) (T) **7.00** The Big Breakfast. **9.00** The Morning Line. (T) **9.30** 4Learning. **12.00** Powerhouse. (T) **12.30** Cheers. (R) (T) **1.00** Cheltenham Festival. Races at 2.00, 2.35, 3.15 and 3.55. (T) **4.30** Countdown. Word game. (T) (S)

5.00 Richard & Judy. (T)

6.00 Eden. The past couple of days' events. (T)

6.30 Hollyoaks. Mandy takes a driving lesson. (T)

7.00 Channel 4 News. (T)

7.40 Cheltenham Gold Cup Re-Run. (T) (R)

7.55 £25 Equals MC Squared. (T)

8.00 Brookside. Marty appeals to Max for help; Jimmy lands in hospital following his arrest and Rachel keeps quiet about her new job. (T)

8.30 Driven. The team visit the Geneva Motorshow to bring news of the hottest new cars. (T)

9.00 Dispatches. How a lack of proper controls is allowing financial, physical and even sexual abuse to take place in Britain's mosques. (T)

10.00 Friends. Joey plans to kiss Janine. (T) (R)

10.30 Trigger Happy TV. (T)

11.35 The Estate Agents. Last in series. (T)

Channel 5

6.00 Sunrise. (S) **6.30** Milkshake!: Dappledown Farm. **6.55** Nosey. (S) **7.00** Happy Monsters. (R) (S) **7.15** Little Antics. (S) **7.30** Tickle, Patch and Friends. (R) (S) **8.00** Bear in the Big Blue House. (R) (S) **8.30** Beachcomber Bay. (S) **9.00** Havakazoo. (R) (S) **9.30** House Doctor. (R) (T) (S) **10.00** The Wright Stuff. (S) **11.00** TJ Hooker. (R) (T) (S) **12.00** 5 News. (T) **12.30** Home and Away. (R) (T) (S) **1.00** Family Affairs. (R) (T) (S) **1.30** The Oprah Winfrey Show. (S) **2.20** Open House with Gloria Hunniford. (T) (S) **3.35 FILM:** The Whistle Blower (1986). (T)

5.30 5 News; Weather. (T)

6.00 Home and Away. (T) (S)

6.30 Family Affairs. Claire is disappointed by Tom's lack of romantic interest; (T) (S) 5 News Update.

7.00 The Pepsi Chart. Performances by Blue and Darren Hayes. (S)

7.30 5 News; Weather. (T)

8.00 Libel. Kelvin MacKenzie explores the world of High Court libel cases, including incidents involving famous faces such as Elton John, Mohammed Al-Fayed and Gillian Taylforth; (T) (S) 5 News

9.00 FILM: Fatherland (1994). A journalist and a detective attempt to topple the Third Reich in an alternative 1960s where Hitler won the war. (T)

11.05 G-String Divas. (S) (R)

11.45 Johnathan Pearce's Football Night. (S)

Five activities task

Task 4: Crosswords

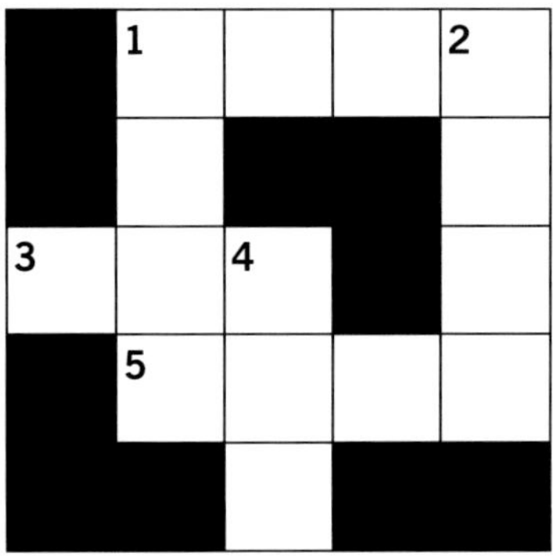

ACROSS

1 This is knocked into wood with a hammer
3 Frozen water
5 Edge of the pavement near the road

DOWN

1 It joins your head to your body
2 A baby sheep
4 A long fish shaped like a snake

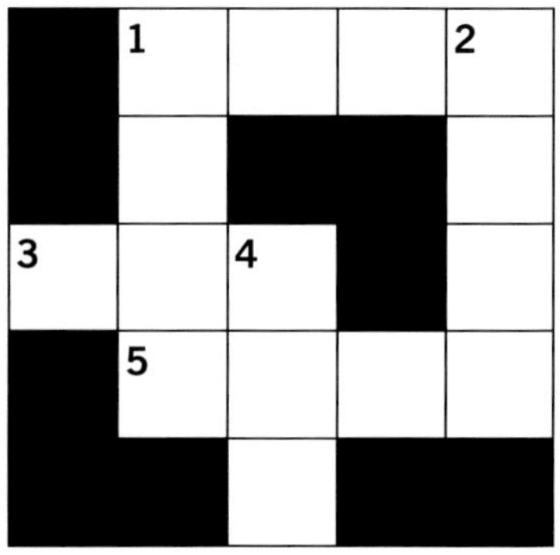

ACROSS

1 Another word for tins
3 Not thin
5 You do this to letters in a pillar box

DOWN

1 Strike hands together
2 He was hit with a bullet
4 Opposite of 'bottom'

Task 5: Degraded Letters

Directions: The figures below represent parts of letters. Complete them by adding lines, curves, or both to each figure. They will spell words from each of the named categories.

1 WEATHER

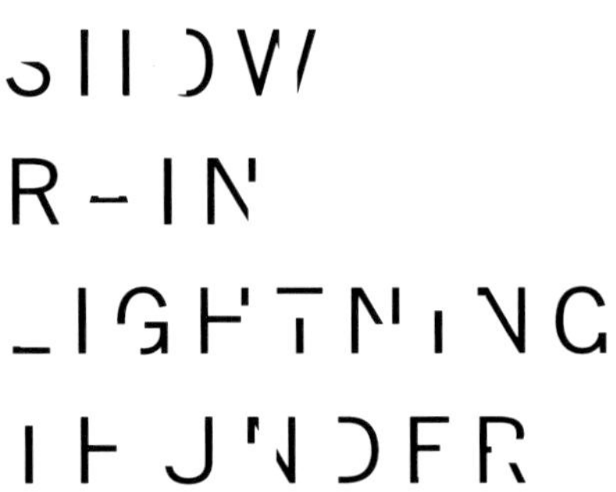

2 SPORTS

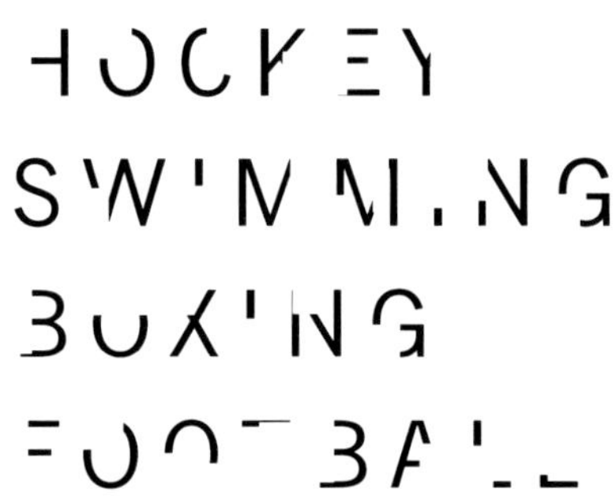

Discuss how you coped with the five activities tasks. Did you follow the rules and succeed? What strategies did you use?

How did you find this exercise? Easy ☐ OK ☐ Quite difficult ☐ Very difficult ☐

Action plans

How difficult do you think you will find this exercise? Easy ☐ OK ☐ Quite difficult ☐ Very difficult ☐

Instruction

Choose one of the following tasks, and write out at least 10 steps required for the completion of the task:

1 Putting up a shelf in the kitchen
2 Mending a puncture on a child's bicycle
3 Arranging a day trip to Paris

Task

What strategies did you use?

How did you find this exercise? Easy ☐ OK ☐ Quite difficult ☐ Very difficult ☐

EXERCISE 17

Who will survive?

How difficult do you think you will find this exercise? Easy ☐ OK ☐ Quite difficult ☐ Very difficult ☐

Instruction

Imagine a nuclear disaster has occurred, and the world as we know it has been destroyed. However, YOU have the power to save six people, who will survive and hopefully continue the human race. Out of the 12 people below, which six would you entrust with the future of mankind? Put a tick next to the six you would save. Carry out this task in groups, or individually.

1 Dr Jane Smith, 29, GP, mother of two, likes painting and gardening.
2 Errol, 22, unemployed, history of car theft and minor drug abuse, played basketball at school.
3 Jenny, 21, fashion model, long history of anorexia and some drug abuse.
4 James, 23, medical student, plays tennis, enjoys amateur dramatics, good sense of humour.
5 Marcus, 45, artist, unmarried, long history of heroin dependency.
6 Dr Len Murray, 75-year-old retired brain surgeon, plays piano.
7 Susie Lee, 27, Chinese but speaks good English, married with one child, physicist.
8 Jim Wright, 36, father, computer consultant, captain of local soccer team, smoker.
9 Sarah, 26, single parent, works as a caterer, enjoys organising parties.
10 Veronica, 53, housewife, mother of five, good cook.
11 David, 28, young farmer, plays soccer, has a schizophrenic cousin.
12 Mary, 25, psychologist, lesbian, enjoys cycling and marathon running.

What are the important variables that you have considered?

How did you find this exercise? Easy ☐ OK ☐ Quite difficult ☐ Very difficult ☐

Sentence sequencing

How difficult do you think you will find this exercise? Easy ☐ OK ☐ Quite difficult ☐ Very difficult ☐

Instruction

Put the following sentences in the correct order to make a story:

A Hannah didn't want her Dad to go into the girls' changing room, as she'd be embarrassed.
B She was getting irritated because he couldn't do it.
C Hannah has a swimming lesson on Thursday evening at 7.30.
D Thankfully, a nice lady who had been in the swimming club for years helped him out.
E Dad struggled to put the swimming cap over her head in the corridor.
F Her mother usually takes her, but tonight her Dad took her.
G This was a problem, as Hannah needed help putting her swimming cap on.

Correct order:

1 ____ **2** ____ **3** ____ **4** ____ **5** ____ **6** ____ **7** ____

What strategies did you use?

Make up your own jumbled story sequence with three sentences. Read it out to the group and they have to sort out the correct order.

How did you find this exercise? Easy ☐ OK ☐ Quite difficult ☐ Very difficult ☐

Planning courses

How difficult do you think you will find this exercise? Easy ☐ OK ☐ Quite difficult ☐ Very difficult ☐

Instruction

You are a busy working parent and would like to take your two children, Jane (aged seven years) and Henry (aged nine years), on sports courses. Jane is interested in trampolining, but has never done it before. Henry is a good swimmer and diver but would like to improve his diving. All the sports facilities are within 5 minutes' walk of each other. The children say that they are quite happy to sit and watch each other carry out their events as long as you buy them a comic and some sweets. You would prefer to carry out both activities on the same day.

➤ On which course would you enrol Jane?

➤ On which course would you enrol Henry?

DIVING

We offer a comprehensive diving award scheme which is structured to develop good basic diving techniques, teach children how to use the springboards and diving platforms safely and effectively.

CENTRAL POOL	TUES	4.00–4.30pm	6+ yrs	Beginners
		4.30–5.00pm	6+ yrs	Beginners
		5.00–5.30pm	6+ yrs	Improvers
		5.30–6.00pm	6+ yrs	Improvers
	WED	6.15–6.50pm	8+ yrs	Begs/Imps
		6.50–7.25pm	8+ yrs	Improvers
		7.25–8.00pm	8+ yrs	Beginners
		8.00–8.30pm	8+ yrs	Beginners
	FRI	4.30–5.00pm	8+ yrs	Beginners
		5.00–5.30pm	8+ yrs	Beginners
		5.30–6.00pm	6+ yrs	Beginners
		6.00–6.30pm	6+ yrs	Improvers
		6.30–7.00pm	6+ yrs	Beginners
	SAT	8.30–9.00am	8+ yrs	Begs/Imps
		9.00–9.30am	8+ yrs	Improvers
		9.35–10.10am	8+ yrs	Begs/Ints
		10.10–10.45am	8+ yrs	Beginners

TENNIS

Our coach will help children develop basic forehand, backhand and serving skills, progressing towards match play skills and tactics.

PALMER PARK	SAT	9.30–10.30am	8–15 yrs	Beginners
	SAT	10.30–11.30am	8–15 yrs	Improvers

BADMINTON

Our badminton coaching scheme caters for all abilities of junior badminton player. Children can work towards badges and certificates from the ESBA scheme.

MEADWAY	MON	5.00–6.00pm	6+ yrs	Begs/Imps
		6.00–7.00pm	6+ yrs	Improvers
		7.00–8.00pm	6+ yrs	Advanced

TRAMPOLINING

The RSL tranpoline programme teaches children the basic bounces at beginner level and gradually develops these into more complex moves, twists & somersaults as children progress through the scheme.

MEADWAY	THURS	5.00–6.00pm	5–8 yrs	Beginners
		6.00–7.00pm	9+ yrs	Beginners
		7.00–8.00pm	Senior	Advanced
	SAT	10.00–11.00am	5–8 yrs	Beginners
		11.00–12noon	9–12 yrs	Begs/Imps
		12.00–1.00pm	13+ yrs	Begs/Imps
SOUTH READING	TUES	5.30–6.30pm	6+ yrs	Mixed Ability
		6.30–7.30pm	8+ yrs	Improvers
		7.30–8.30pm	8+ yrs	Mixed Ability
	FRI	4.00–4.45pm	5–8 yrs	Beginners
		4.45–5.30pm	5–8 yrs	Beginners
		5.30–6.30pm	5–8 yrs	Improvers

What strategies did you use to complete the task?

How did you find this exercise? Easy ☐ OK ☐ Quite difficult ☐ Very difficult ☐

Pros and cons

How difficult do you think you will find this exercise? Easy ☐ OK ☐ Quite difficult ☐ Very difficult ☐

Instruction

Choose topics from the subjects below, and try to list at least three reasons for that particular idea (pros), and as many reasons against (cons). Then make up your own topic to discuss.

Capital punishment	Abortion	Legislation to stop smoking in public
Competitive sport at school	Euthanasia	Sex education in schools
Being a vegetarian	Hitch-hiking	Banning tobacco advertising

Issue	
Pros	Cons
➤	➤
➤	➤
➤	➤

Issue	
Pros	Cons
➤	➤
➤	➤
➤	➤

Issue	
Pros	Cons
➤	➤
➤	➤
➤	➤

How did you find this exercise? Easy ☐ OK ☐ Quite difficult ☐ Very difficult ☐

Positives and negatives

How difficult do you think you will find this exercise? Easy ☐ OK ☐ Quite difficult ☐ Very difficult ☐

Instruction

Write down three positive and three negative aspects to the following situations. There are no right or wrong answers, so use your imagination – stretch your thinking.

You have just won the lottery.	
Positive	Negative
➤	➤
➤	➤
➤	➤

You have sprained your ankle badly and have been instructed not to put weight on it, and to rest in bed for two days.	
Positive	Negative
➤	➤
➤	➤
➤	➤

Think of a situation in your own life – or a decision you have to make – and work out the positives and negatives.	
Positive	Negative
➤	➤
➤	➤
➤	➤

How did you find this exercise? Easy ☐ OK ☐ Quite difficult ☐ Very difficult ☐

Problem-solving

How difficult do you think you will find this exercise? Easy ☐ OK ☐ Quite difficult ☐ Very difficult ☐

Instruction

Identify three possible causes for each of these situations.

Your daily newspaper is not on the step at the usual time.
➤
➤
➤

You cannot find your car in a multi-storey car-park.
➤
➤
➤

Somebody you do not know is knocking at your door.
➤
➤
➤

The dog next door has been barking for a long time.
➤
➤
➤

The light in your room goes out.
➤
➤
➤

How did you find this exercise? Easy ☐ OK ☐ Quite difficult ☐ Very difficult ☐

Describe a diagram

How difficult do you think you will find this exercise? Easy ☐ OK ☐ Quite difficult ☐ Very difficult ☐

Instruction

Draw a diagram in the space below, but do not let your partner see it. Then describe it precisely to your partner or the rest of the group. No questions or gestures are allowed. The partner or group draw the diagram from the instructions given. Compare their pictures with yours. Then change over so they draw a diagram and give you instructions. The aim of the exercise is to give as precise and accurate instructions as possible.

Example of diagrams

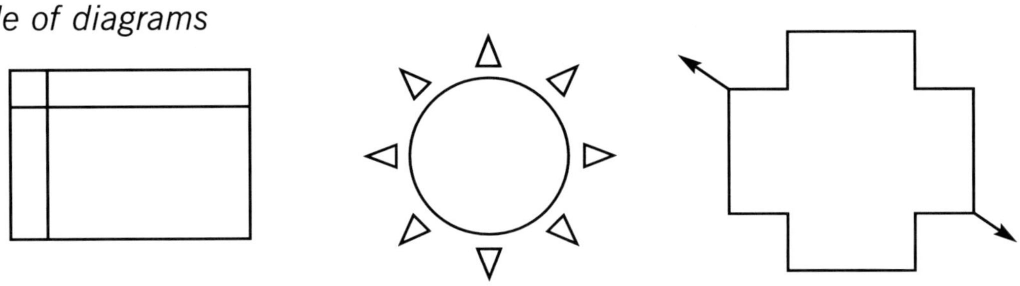

Draw your own diagram

Copy of diagram from instruction

How did you find this exercise? Easy ☐ OK ☐ Quite difficult ☐ Very difficult ☐

Recognising emotions

How difficult do you think you will find this exercise? Easy ☐ OK ☐ Quite difficult ☐ Very difficult ☐

Instruction

Look at the expressions of the people illustrated below. Use one word for each illustration to describe that person's expression.

disgusted	surprised	happy
sad/tearful	bored	thoughtful
furious	worried	vain

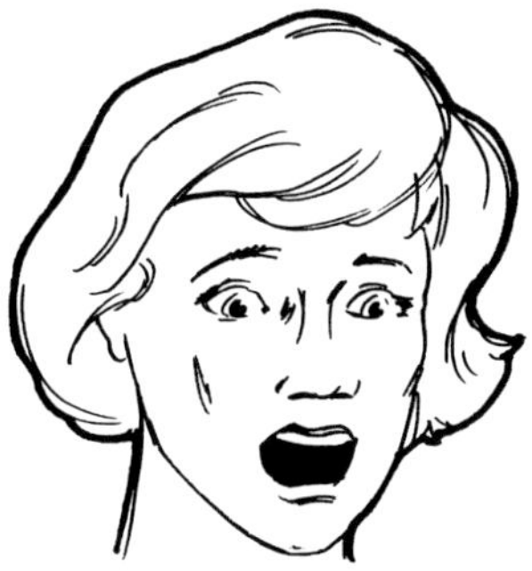

1

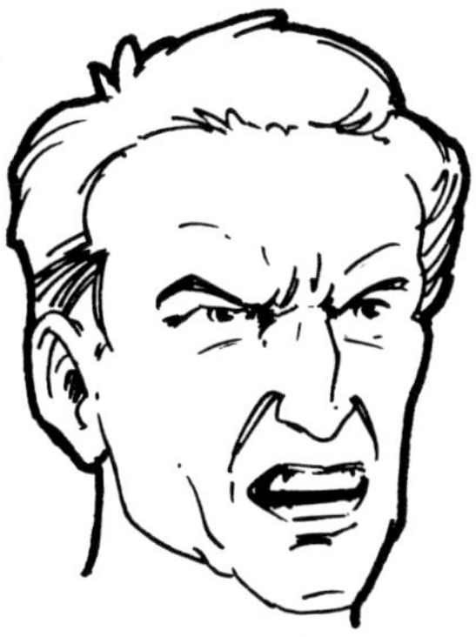

2

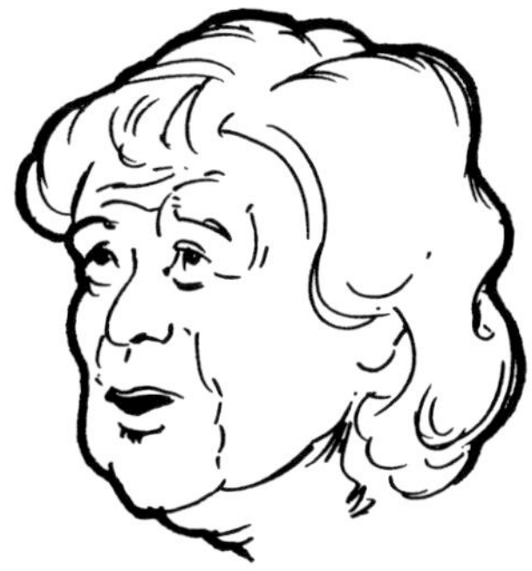

3

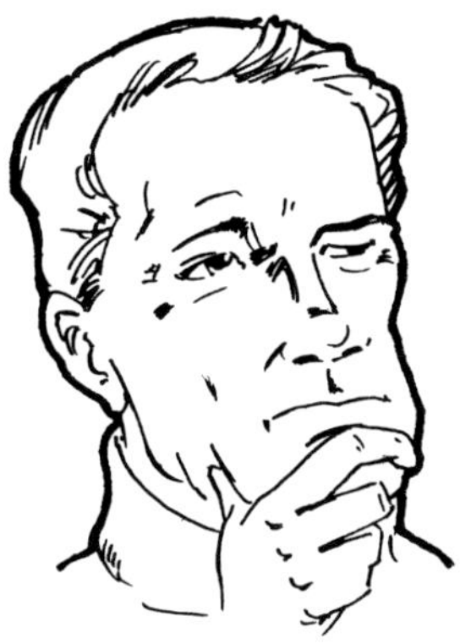

4

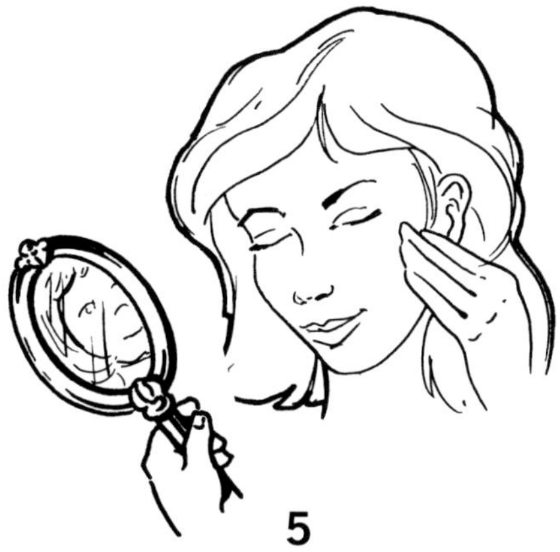

5

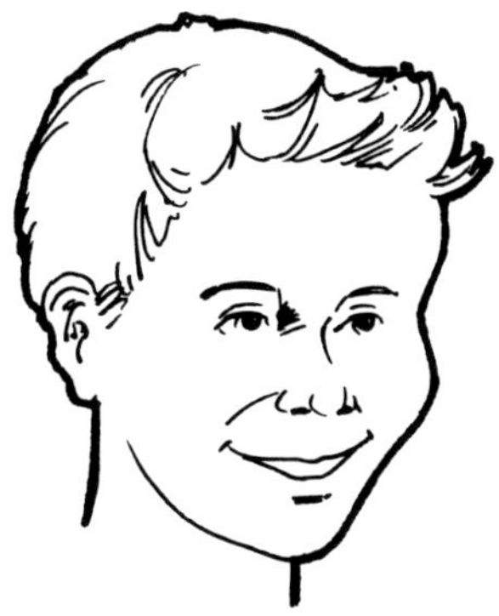

6

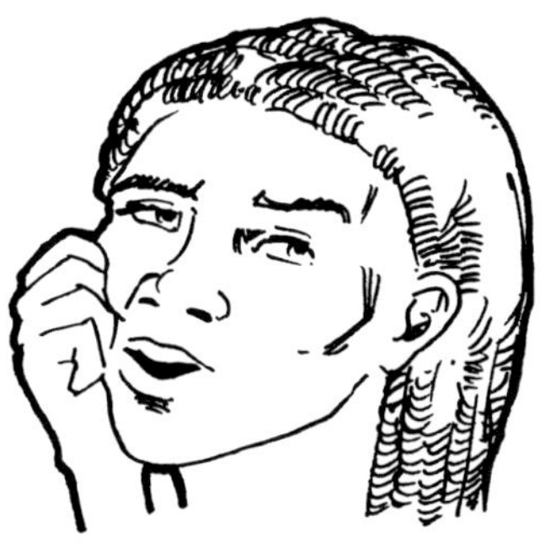

7

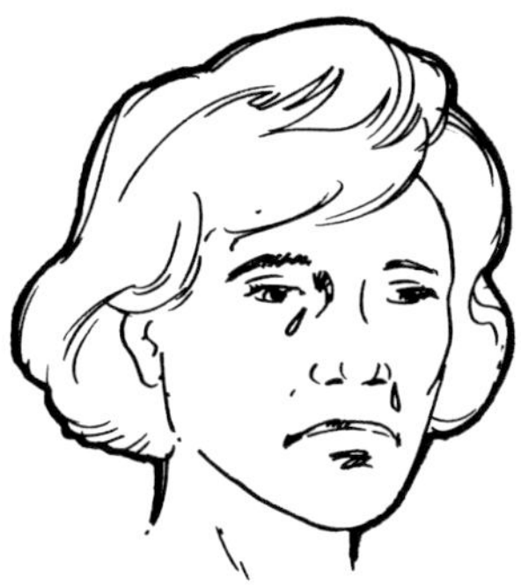

8

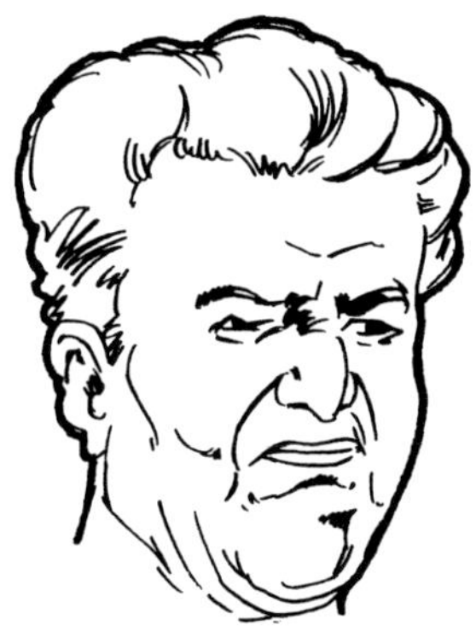

9

How did you find this exercise? Easy ☐ OK ☐ Quite difficult ☐ Very difficult ☐

Plan your busy morning

How difficult do you think you will find this exercise? Easy ☐ OK ☐ Quite difficult ☐ Very difficult ☐

Instruction

Plan your morning by looking at the list of activities you have to complete, and studying the map below.
Then: (1) Fill in your proposed timetable below, using the planner, and arranging the activities in the best possible sequence to make best use of time; (2) Draw your proposed route on the map.

Activities to do:

1 Get money from bank.
2 Take 12-year-old daughter to synchronised swimming – lesson starts at 11am, finishes at 1pm. You don't stay to watch.
3 Go to chemist.
4 Take a load of bags of paper and bottles to the recycling area – the back of your car is fully loaded.
5 Go to supermarket and do weekly shop for a family of three.
6 You leave home at 10.35am and need to get back by 1.30pm – the journey to the Pool takes 10 minutes.

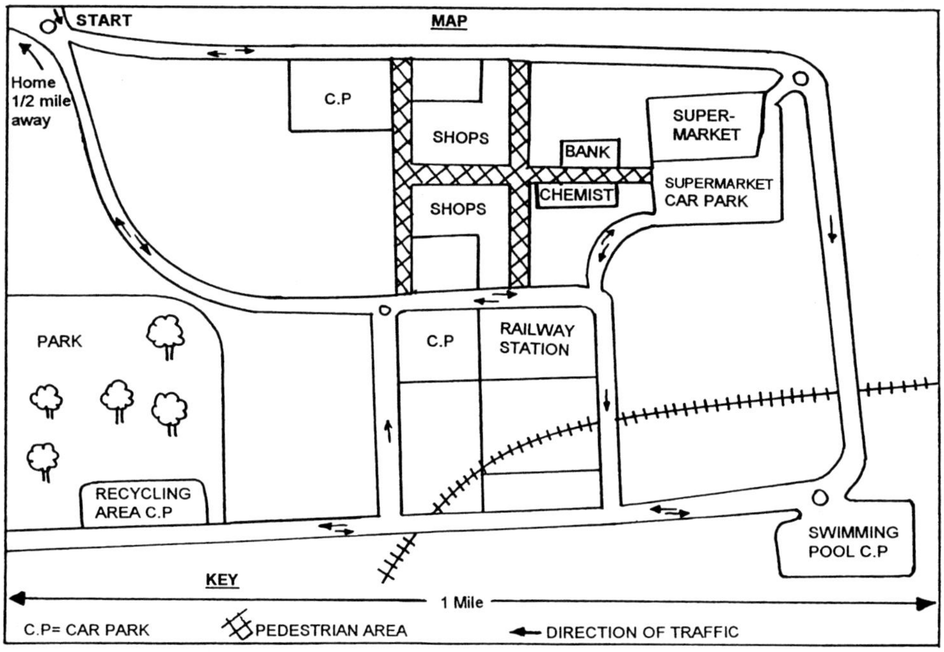

PLANNER
10.30am
10.45
11.00
11.15
11.30
11.45
12.00
12.15pm
12.30
12.45
1.00
1.15
1.30

Identify and discuss which strategies you used to complete this task.

How did you find this exercise? Easy ☐ OK ☐ Quite difficult ☐ Very difficult ☐

EXERCISE 26

Rearrange the pictures 1

How difficult do you think you will find this exercise? Easy ☐ OK ☐ Quite difficult ☐ Very difficult ☐

Instruction

Number each picture in the correct sequence to make a story.

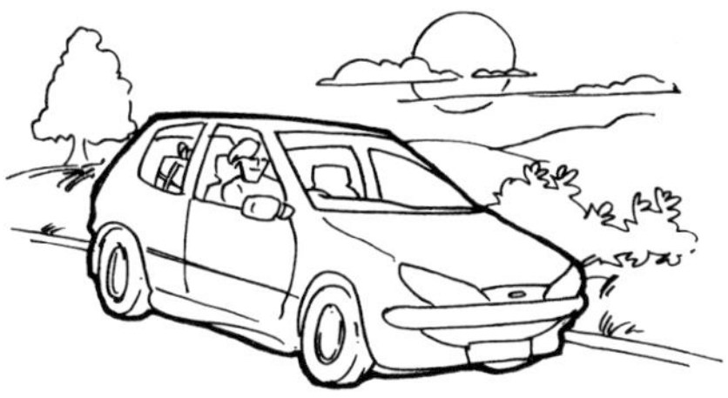

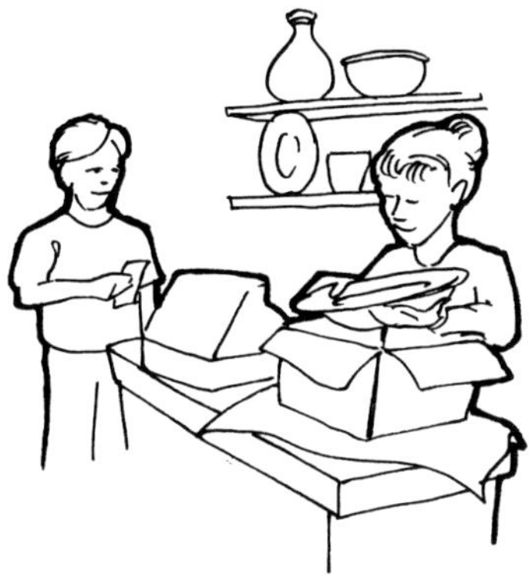

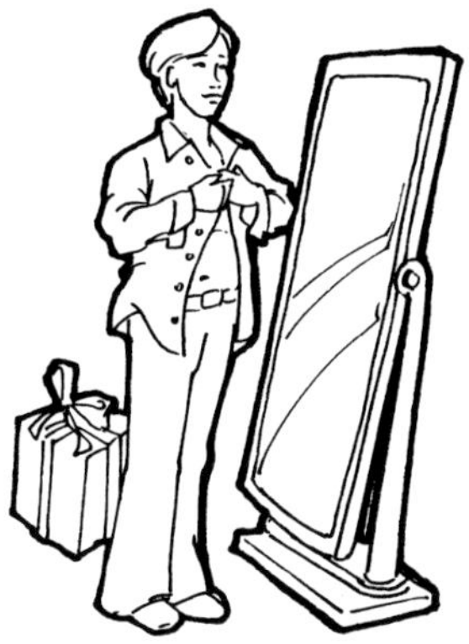

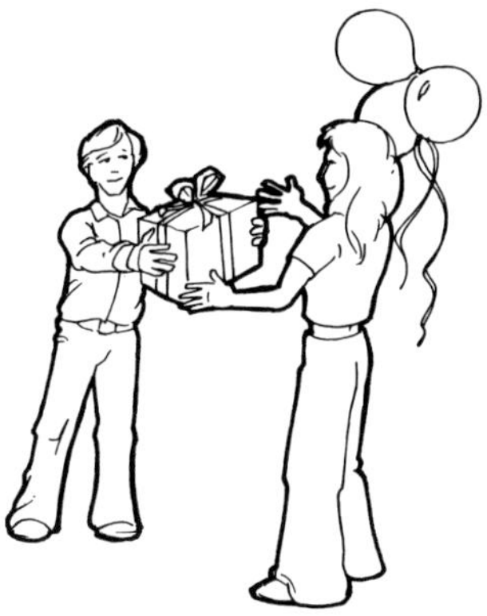

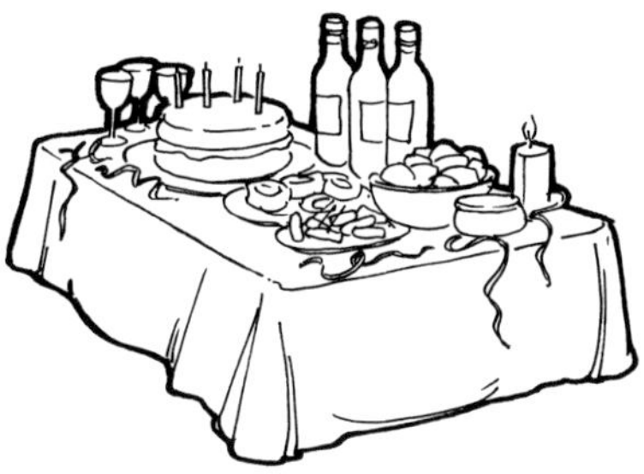

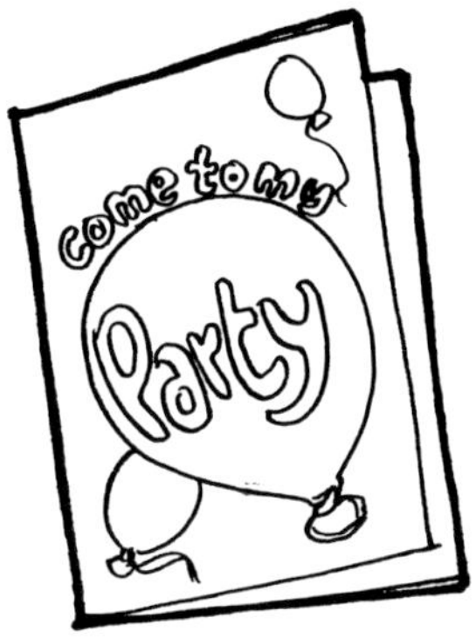

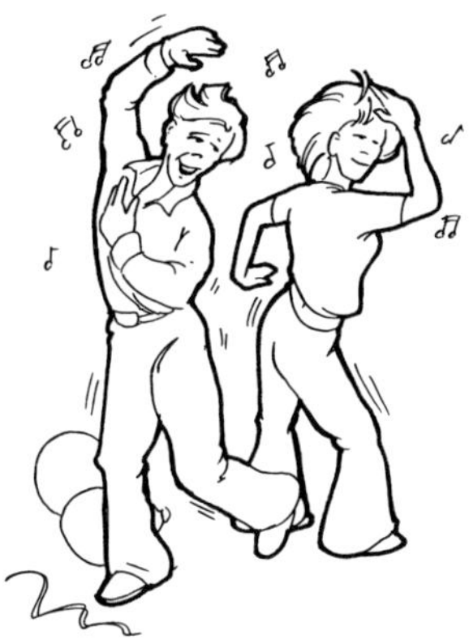

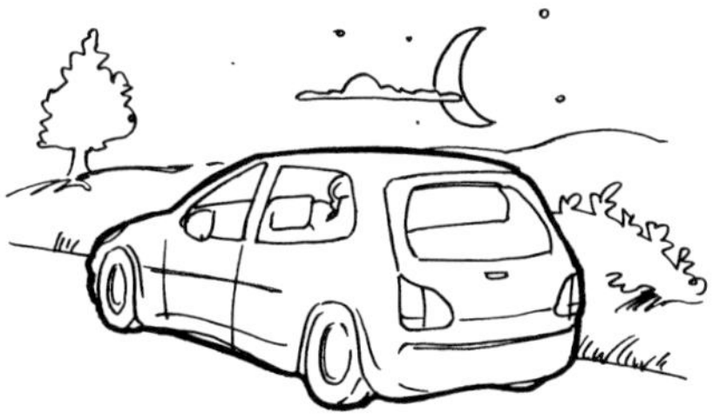

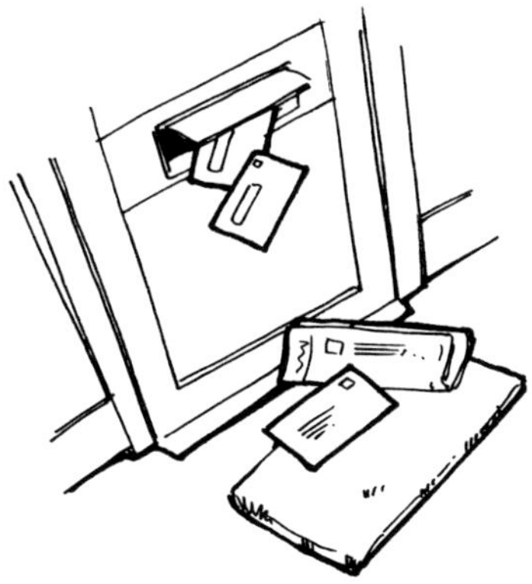

What strategies did you use?

How did you find this exercise? Easy ☐ OK ☐ Quite difficult ☐ Very difficult ☐

Rearrange the pictures 2

How difficult do you think you will find this exercise? Easy ☐ OK ☐ Quite difficult ☐ Very difficult ☐

Instruction

Number each picture in the correct sequence to make a story.

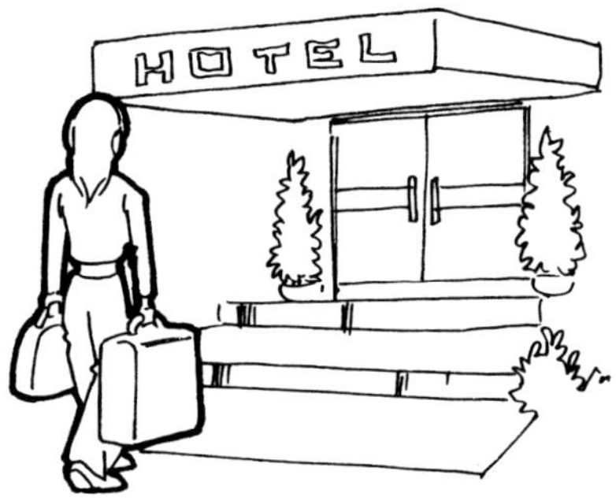

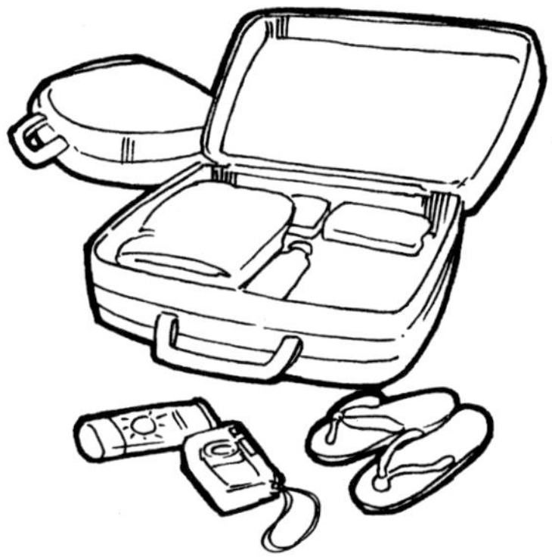

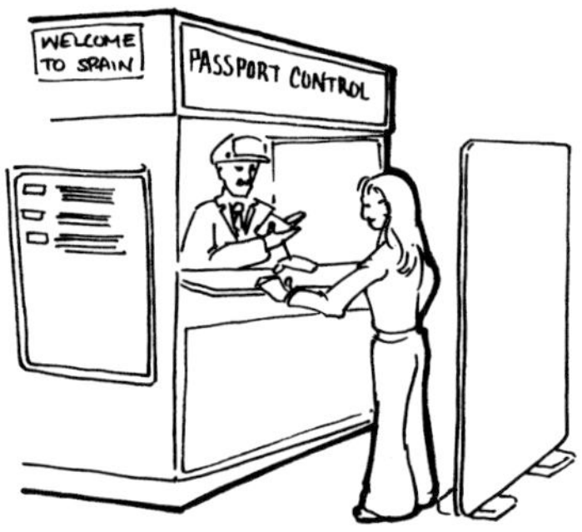

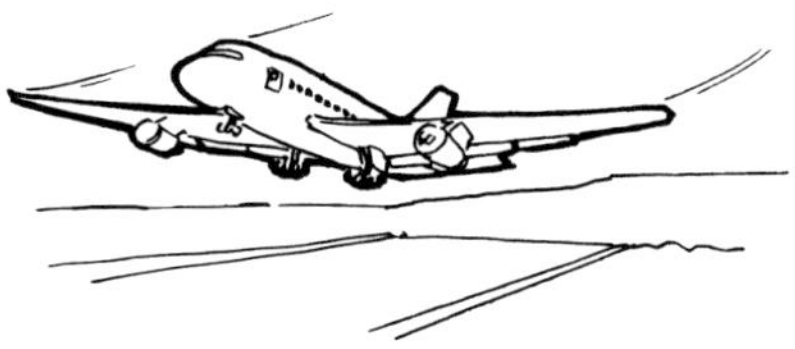

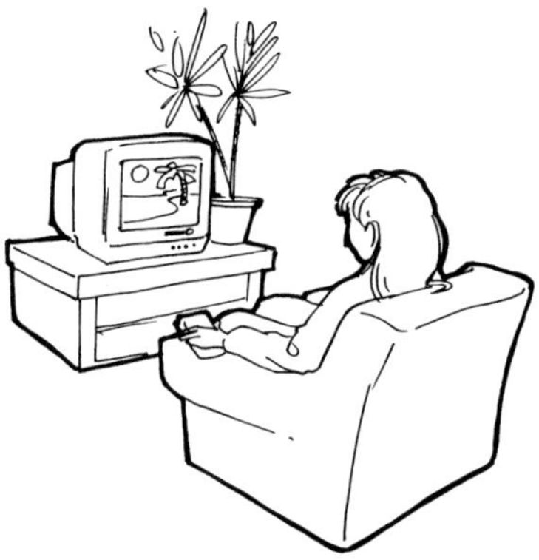

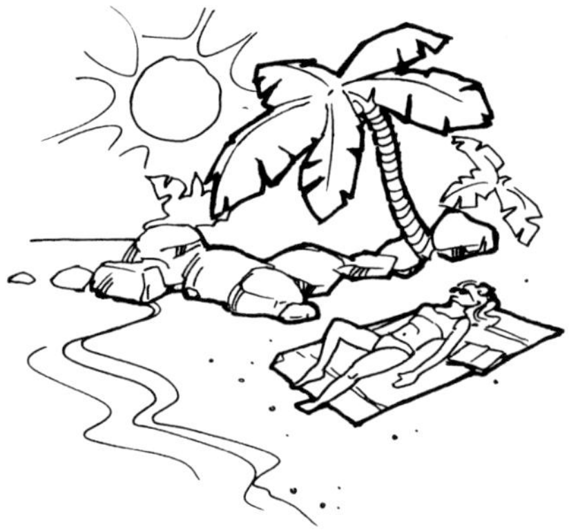

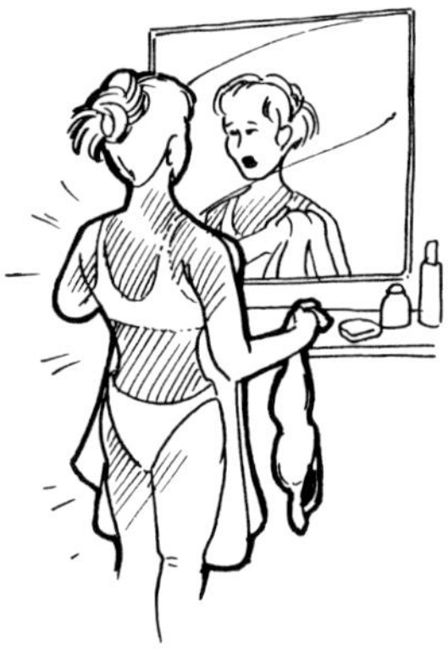

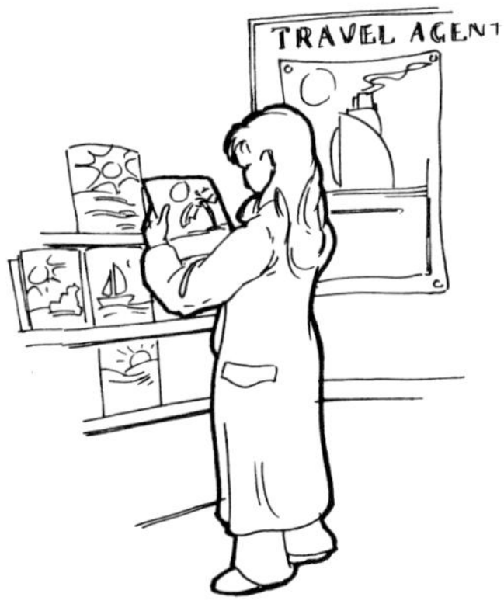

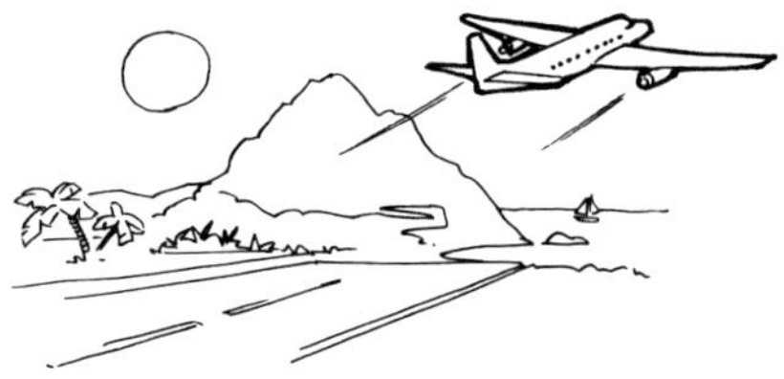

What strategies did you use?

How did you find this exercise? Easy ☐ OK ☐ Quite difficult ☐ Very difficult ☐

EXERCISE 28

Rearrange the pictures 3

How difficult do you think you will find this exercise? Easy ☐ OK ☐ Quite difficult ☐ Very difficult ☐

Instruction

Number each picture in the correct sequence to make a story.

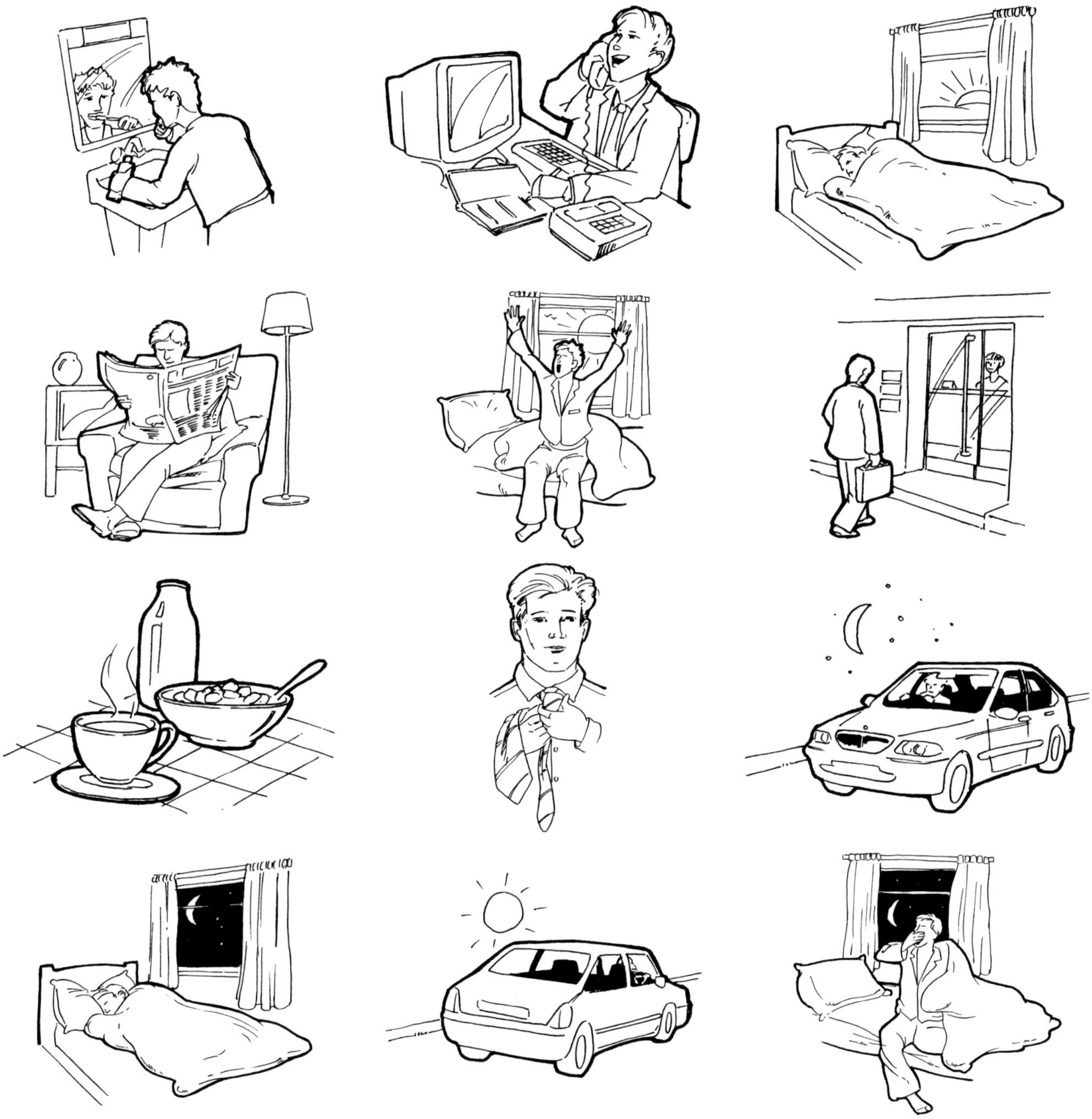

What strategies did you use?

How did you find this exercise? Easy ☐ OK ☐ Quite difficult ☐ Very difficult ☐

What's the headline?

How difficult do you think you will find this exercise? Easy ☐ OK ☐ Quite difficult ☐ Very difficult ☐

Instruction

Below are a number of brief news stories, which all have short headlines of no more than six words. Make up your own headlines that are both eye-catching and give an accurate summary of the news story.

Example (5 words) **Woman found dead in river**	3 words
Detectives started a murder inquiry last night after the body of a woman was found in a river near a marina at Great Yarmouth, Norfolk. Police said she had been strangled.	A swastika was daubed on a rabbi's lectern by vandals who smashed windows, defaced religious artifacts and left excrement in an attack on Finsbury Park synagogue, North London, at the weekend, it was revealed yesterday.
5 words	6 words
Greece shut all schools three days early for the Orthodox Easter holiday yesterday in an attempt to stem the spread of a flu-like virus which is believed to have killed three people and infected 29 in less than a week. *Reuters, Athens.*	Human remains found in a tiger shark caught off the coast of New South Wales have been identified as those of a 52-year-old Sydney man swept out to sea while fishing from rocks 90 miles north of the city on April 2. *AP, Sydney.*
6 words	5 words
Three men and two women will appear today at the Sheriff's court in Dingwall, near Inverness, charged with breach of the peace and vandalism after GM crops in a field at Munlochy in the Highlands were destroyed.	Leeds education chiefs were investigating yesterday after pupils at Saint Joseph's community high school were 'considerably distressed' by a teacher with a starting pistol. The gun was to have been used in a physics lesson.

What strategies did you use to carry out this task?

How did you find this exercise? Easy ☐ OK ☐ Quite difficult ☐ Very difficult ☐

Wedding reception venues

How difficult do you think you will find this exercise? Easy ☐ OK ☐ Quite difficult ☐ Very difficult ☐

Instruction

You are trying to pick a venue for a wedding reception. You have identified five requirements, now choose which one venue fits the bill.

- Must be able to seat 100 people
- Must be near Reading
- Must have varied menu
- Total cost no more than £1,500
- Preferably in a memorable location

1 The Rainbow Inn is available as a conference centre or function room. It is located beside the River Thames in Marlow, and can seat 130 people. There is an excellent choice of four set menus. The cost is £1,800, including food.	
2 The Warwick Arms. This historic oak-beamed pub in Henley was frequented by the poet Shelley. It has facilities for small functions of about 90 people. The venue may be hired for £1,200, and our nationally renowned chef is available for discussion of your menu choices.	
3 Reading Town Hall has a large function room where it is possible to seat 200 people beneath the old red-brick arches and stained glass windows. The room costs £1,500, including the waiters and master of ceremonies, and the menu has three choices for each course.	
4 The Hilton Hotel in Brighton has a well equipped conference centre that is also suitable for family or office events. It is priced at £800, plus a choice of menus to be negotiated with the hotel caterer.	
5 Bancroft Hall near Tilehurst, Reading, offers its historic Tudor barn as the ideal setting for parties of up to 120 people, and wedding receptions. The room costs £900 with a set menu.	

What strategies did you use to do this task?

How did you find this exercise? Easy ☐ OK ☐ Quite difficult ☐ Very difficult ☐

Renting an apartment

How difficult do you think you will find this exercise? Easy ☐ OK ☐ Quite difficult ☐ Very difficult ☐

Instruction

You are looking to rent an apartment. You have identified five requirements, now choose which of the following apartments would be most suitable.

- You can afford to pay £450 per month rent
- Must be fully furnished
- You have a cat who likes to go outside
- You have a teenage daughter
- You have a grand piano

	Yes/No
1 This spacious ground-floor apartment is available for £600 per month. It has a fully fitted kitchen, large sitting room, two bedrooms and luxurious bathroom. Close to shops and station.	
2 £320 per month! Ideal for a young professional, this unfurnished ground-floor apartment in a large Victorian house has one double bedroom and a spacious sitting room with French windows leading to a delightful small garden.	
3 This second-floor apartment in a purpose-built block has two bedrooms and a compact kitchen and sitting room. Available immediately, fully furnished – £100 per week. Not suitable for an elderly person (no lift).	
4 Available from September, a two-bedroomed ground-floor apartment with an exceptionally spacious sitting room/dining room. Available part-furnished or fully furnished at £110 per week. Large communal garden. Close to shops and bus routes.	
5 Only £450 per month, this beautifully decorated and fully furnished first-floor apartment has two bedrooms and forms part of a seventeenth-century farmhouse. Its rooms are small, but full of character.	

What strategies did you use to complete the task?

How did you find this exercise? Easy ☐ OK ☐ Quite difficult ☐ Very difficult ☐

PART III

Emotional Adjustment

Awareness Skills

INFORMATION SHEETS

AWARENESS SKILLS EXERCISES

Awareness skills questionnaire

Name ______________________ Date ______________

This questionnaire assesses your level of awareness. Read each of the statements, and mark the box that best describes your beliefs at present. Then ask someone who knows you well to complete the questionnaire and fill in the independent scorer column. Compare the two columns.

Scoring Agree = 2 Partially agree = 1 Disagree = 0

Question	**Score**					
	Self-score			Independent scorer		
	Agree	Partially agree	Disagree	Agree Agree	Partially agree	Disagree
1 I have noticed that I have some problems with my memory and concentration.						
2 I have noticed that my temperament is different, eg, I lose my temper more quickly, or I am more 'laid back'.						
3 I have noticed that my ability to communicate with others is not as good as it was.						
4 I feel that my life has changed in some ways since my injury.						
5 I do have problems with organising and planning.						
6 My relationships with people have altered since my injury.						
7 I am not as competent and efficient as I used to be.						
8 I tend to make more careless errors than I did before my injury.						
9 I cannot do all the things that I used to do because of my injury.						
10 The injury was a turning point in my life, and life will never be the same again.						
TOTAL SCORE						

INTERPRETATION

Discrepancy between self-score and independent score

5–20: It may be that you are not fully aware of your difficulties. Work carefully through this Awareness section.

How relevant did you find this sheet? Very ☐ Slightly ☐ Not very ☐

Understanding awareness

Our ability for self-reflection, to be aware of our strengths and weaknesses, and to monitor our effects on others, is known as insight or awareness and is one of the highest human abilities. Apes are the only other animals, apart from humans, that can use a mirror and reflect on themselves.

People who have had a brain injury invariably have reduced awareness. There is a tendency to underestimate difficulties and to overestimate abilities. One study found that seven years after injury, 30 per cent of relatives said that the person with brain injury 'refused to admit to difficulties'.

Awareness is a common problem following brain injury, because of damage to vital parts of the frontal lobe area of the brain – particularly the right side. Impaired self-awareness is directly related to extent of loss of consciousness.

A variety of factors can add to impaired awareness:

(a) If the individual is in either a coma or a state of post-traumatic amnesia, he is not able to be fully aware of what is happening; whereas relatives and clinicians see the patient close to death or severely injured, and appreciate the severity of the situation.

(b) The person with brain injury usually notices tangible physical impairments such as being unable to walk, more readily than intangible, subtle, cognitive, or emotional impairments.

(c) People with brain injury are often in a hospital environment, where cognitive skills are not tested. It is only when they go back home or to work that they realise the problems.

(d) People with brain injury have few rituals to help them come to terms with the changes and losses. There are no funerals, court hearings, or leaving parties, so they have no chance to grieve and emotionally adjust.

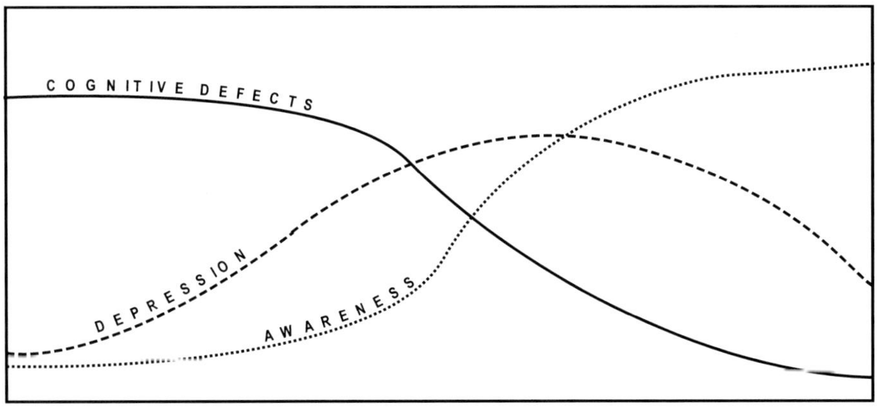

STAGES OF RECOVERY

It has been suggested that there are stages of recovery, and that as cognitive deficits – such as memory and thinking – improve, awareness also improves. This improvement in awareness is often accompanied by an increase in anxiety and depression.

Understanding awareness

It has been suggested that there are three types of awareness deficit:

(a) **Pure neurological inability, or anosagnosia** (*a* = without; *gnosis* = knowledge; *nosis* = disease). In its purest form, this can be a lack of awareness of, for example, paralysis, blindness, or a spatial neglect. This is usually due to damage in the back part (posterior) of the right hemisphere.

(b) **Lack of awareness due to cognitive deficits.** Global cognitive problems, such as memory, attention and executive skills impairments mean that the person cannot piece together and appreciate their deficits. When confronted, the person with this kind of awareness problem typically displays an emotional response, usually showing 'heightened concern'.

(c) **Denial.** This can be conscious or unconscious, but is a response – largely a 'psychological defence mechanism'- where the person does not want to know or accept the problem because it is too painful to face. When the person with denial is confronted, their response is often that of anger and arousal. They may tend to rationalise, minimalise, or blame the environment for difficulties, rather than accepting the reality.

There appear to be different levels of awareness deficit. At the basic level, there is 'intellectual awareness', where the person can describe their difficulties, but does not do anything about them. A slightly higher level is 'emergent awareness', where the individual can recognise problems without feedback from others, and may even attempt to correct them there and then. The highest level is 'anticipatory awareness', where the person anticipates that problems are going to happen, because of their deficits, and make deliberate compensatory plans.

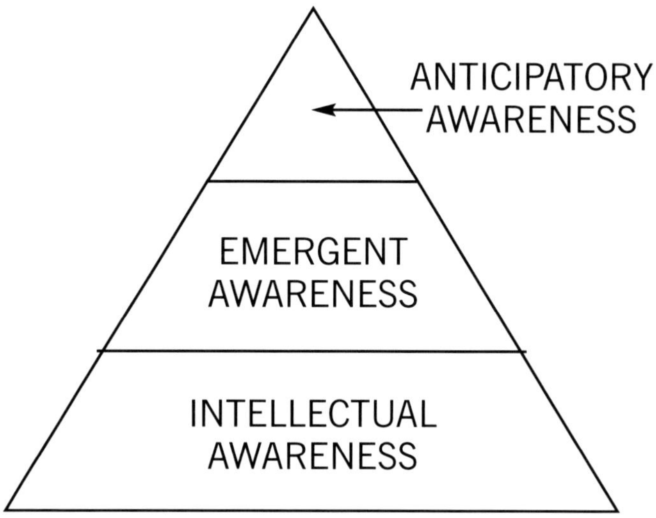

1. What factors affect levels of awareness?
2. Describe the three different types of 'awareness difficulty'.
3. Describe the three different levels of awareness difficulty.
4. Which level of awareness do you think you have?

How relevant did you find this sheet? Very ☐ Slightly ☐ Not very ☐

Ways of improving awareness

Timing. It is important to be aware that a judgement needs to be made about the best time to provide these interventions – for example, provision of information about long-term disability at a very early stage, when the client's everyday memory is not working well, would not be a good idea.

Education. Clinicians should give as much information as possible about the nature of the brain injury, including the more subtle, hidden aspects. Provide books and pamphlets, send copies of reports, show scans, and encourage the involvement of the brain-injured person and relatives.

Psychological checklists/test results/ self-rating scales. Feedback of psychological tests, results or scores on checklists or rating scales is useful.

Videotaping. Video feedback in this form is often 'concrete' and difficult to disagree with. It is also easier to view performance after the situation has finished, rather than during it, since this involves less processing capacity.

Working in groups. Meeting other people in the same boat or seeing other people's deficits when in a group situation can make it easier for people to accept that they too might have those problems.

Feedback. Sensitive, honest non-critical feedback in everyday life is vital, but sometimes may be painful to accept.

Planned failure or behavioural experiments. We all learn from our mistakes. Sometimes failing can be helpful, as long as there is emotional support and help, so that it is not too negative an experience.

Individual Psychotherapy. Adjustment counselling over a period of time can help in the process of understanding oneself better.

Rehabilitation games and exercises. Exercises that focus on an area of specific change or deficit, such as memory, executive ability or even awareness itself, can help to lead the client into thinking more about their problem and their new situation.

What particular strategies or interventions have been most helpful to you in gaining awareness of your difficulties?

How relevant did you find this sheet? Very ☐ Slightly ☐ Not very ☐

Emotional changes following brain injury

Anxiety. People are often more easily confused, worry about their ability to carry out everyday activities, and worry about how they will improve and cope with the future.

Depression. In traumatic brain injury and stroke, depression often develops when improvement slows down. It is a recognised stage in the process of adjustment, and seems to occur independently of severity or type of disability.

Emotional lability. This refers to a lack, or loosening, of control of emotions. People often experience extreme and exaggerated emotions that fluctuate wildly. They may break down in tears at a sad news item on the television, or looking at old photographs. A few minutes later the tears may have dried, and they may be laughing. This symptom has been called 'emotional incontinence'.

Emotional flattening or blunting. Sometimes people experience a flattening of their emotional state, and no longer experience the same emotional highs and lows as before their injury. This is a difficult change for partners and carers to live with, because temperamentally the individual has become a very different person.

Disinhibition and lowered tolerance. After a brain injury people often experience a lowered tolerance of frustration, with a tendency to anger much more quickly. The previous emotional controls are lost, and if they feel irritated, they tend to express it directly. Angry outbursts are often very explosive, but short-lived. People may express their thoughts directly, whereas previously they would have been more diplomatic. They are often described as being like Jekyll and Hyde!

Lack of insight. People are not always fully aware of their disability. They may attempt to walk, even though they are unable to do so, or may say 'I'm going back to my old job', even though they have significant problems with thinking and memory.

Bereavement reaction. The process of bereavement occurs with any major loss, including disability due to brain injury. Both the brain-injured person and their relatives go through a process of bereavement. There are various stages in this process which involve: (1) initial shock and perhaps denial; followed by (2) anger and disorganisation; often followed by (3) depression, as the reality of the loss sinks in; then followed by (4) reorganisation and acceptance. This process can take months or a number of years, and may not necessarily occur in this order.

What emotional changes have you experienced since your injury?

How relevant did you find this sheet? Very ☐ Slightly ☐ Not very ☐

Emotions experienced by carers and relatives

Anxiety. Initial anxiety is very common, because the relative does not know what is going to happen and often feels completely out of control. This combination of worrying about the brain injured person, and coping with the everyday stresses is often very tiring, and can lead to symptoms of stress and anxiety.

Depression. This often develops after a certain amount of recovery has taken place, when the carer realises that the changes and disabilities due to the brain injury are likely to be permanent. The hopeful optimism of the early stages of recovery is replaced by a realism that is often accompanied by depressed mood.

Bereavement. Just like the brain injured person, the carer must go through a grieving process that involves shock, denial, disorganisation, anger, depressed mood, sadness, and then reorganisation and acceptance.

Add your own:

Ways of coping for carers and partners

1. Understand more about the problems related to the brain injury, and the relevant symptoms.
2. Talk to others about your feelings, anxieties and worries. Get it out; do not bottle it up.
3. Allow yourself to feel what you feel. Do not 'sweep it under the carpet'.
4. Look after yourself physically; eat well, and ensure that you allow yourself sufficient sleep and relaxation.
5. Try not to withdraw from the company of others: carry on with work, normal hobbies and social activities if possible.
6. Try to make contact with others in a similar position, and discuss similarities and ways of coping.
7. **Add your own:**

> 1. What emotional changes have you experienced since the injury?
> 2. How can you cope with these changes?

How relevant did you find this sheet? Very ☐ Slightly ☐ Not very ☐

Understanding apathy after brain injury

I don't give a damn about apathy
- Groucho Marx

Apathy is a lack of goal-directed behaviour: a loss or impairment of the power or will to execute what is in the mind. There is often difficulty in initiating and sustaining purposeful action, and a poverty of spontaneous action. There is no lack of power in the muscular system, and frequently no lack of desire to reach the end result, but there is a problem in translating that intention or desire into action. This is different from dyspraxia, which is characterised by an inability to carry out specific motor activities due to impairment of cognition and planned movement.

The brain-injured person may spend long periods of time just sitting in front of the television, whereas before their injury they were always on the go. They may not arrange or plan things, and appear to just drift through life. One man said, 'I want to do a thousand things but never get around to doing any.'

The three components of goal-directed behaviour, which are lacking in people with apathy, are:

(a) Having an idea, setting a goal and then breaking it down into achievable steps.
(b) Initiating, or starting, the first step and staying focused – avoiding distraction.
(c) The drive or desire to complete the action – to be really concerned about outcome.

It is important to distinguish apathy from depression. In depression, the brain-injured person socially withdraws, experiences feelings of concern and does not enjoy activities that previously gave pleasure; whereas in primary apathy there is largely indifference and lack of concern.

Neural circuits in the frontal lobes have been associated with motivation and apathy. Interruptions in these circuits probably result in a problem with the production of certain neurotransmitters, such as dopamine.

Ways of coping with apathy

Recognise the problem. It is important to explain the concept of apathy to the family members, as it may help prevent brain-injured people being blamed or criticised for their apparent disinterest and unresponsiveness to well-meaning efforts at rehabilitation. It is important to recognise that the person is not depressed. GPs with little experience of brain injury might often misdiagnose depression when the primary diagnosis is apathy.

Understanding apathy after brain injury

Lower your expectations. If a person has apathy as a result of brain injury, their lifestyle is going to be different – their needs are different.

Break down activities into small steps, to avoid overwhelming the individual. For example, in the morning you could say 'Get yourself dressed.'; then later on say, 'Let's have breakfast.', and then later again say, 'Come with me to the supermarket.' If this was all given at the same time in one sentence, the brain-injured person could easily become overwhelmed.

Engage in activities that the brain-injured person previously enjoyed or was good at.

At times be firm with the person with the brain injury, saying 'We are going to …' rather than 'Do you want to …' Or give the person a choice between two desirable activities.

Reinforce certain desired activities and withdraw rewards for undesirable activities. For example, 'If you get up and go to the shop, I'll make you a cooked breakfast,', rather than bringing the person a cup of tea in bed. Incentives can influence performance, although the underlying motivation can still remain untouched.

Use external cues, such as verbal reminders; or prompts, such as alarm calls. Then gradually withdraw these cues and allow the person to rely on their own internally generated cues. The person needs to be encouraged towards independence as far as possible – to enhance self-esteem.

Structure the day, and try to get into a regular routine. The more regular the routine, the less the brain injured person will have to rely on impaired motivation and executive skills. If the brain-injured person is left with a completely unstructured day, there is a stronger possibility that secondary problems may develop, such as depression, anxiety or confusion.

Encourage involvement in support groups, such as Headway, as this leads to stimulation and encouragement.

> **1** What is apathy?
> **2** In what ways does apathy differ from depression?
> **3** In what ways can you help somebody who suffers from apathy after brain-injury?

How relevant did you find this sheet? Very ☐ Slightly ☐ Not very ☐

Disinhibition and inappropriate behaviour

Disinhibition, or reduced behavioural control, is a major problem after brain injury, and often means that the person is more impulsive and irritable, expressing their feelings, thoughts and opinions without carefully weighing up the consequences. One client said he found that he 'spoke first and thought later'.

The consequence of this is that the person might have impaired social judgement, be over talkative, and say embarrassing things to people. They might also have a very 'short fuse' to their temper and have angry outbursts, often described as being like Jeykll and Hyde – one minute being calm; the next just exploding in rage, and then being calm again.

Disinhibition is often associated with loss of awareness, so the person has no real appreciation that their behaviour is inappropriate and therefore makes no effort to change.

Being disinhibited is somewhat like being a young child, or having a few alcoholic drinks. As the child grows, they learn to control impulses, and this is likely to result in the gradual development of neural pathways in areas of the frontal lobes. Disinhibition is thought to be due to damage to those neural pathways in the frontal lobes.

Ways for the brain-injured person to cope with disinhibition

- Recognise and accept that you have this difficulty – don't blame others. Look for ways of compensating.
- Train yourself to deliberately 'stop and think', and 'step back' before impulsively rushing into something, or saying something you might regret later. Try counting to 10 before acting.
- Keep a record or a diary sheet to identify situations where you think you have been disinhibited. Are you more disinhibited in particular situations? What are the triggers? Knowing this can help you 'put the brakes on' next time you are in that kind of situation.
- Ask other people whom you trust to give you feedback – to tell you when you are being disinhibited, or a 'bit over the top'.
- Apologise to people, and attempt to explain your difficulty.

1 What is disinhibition?
2 Give one practical example of a situation where you might have been disinhibited.
3 Suggest two practical ways of coping with disinhibition.

How relevant did you find this sheet? Very ☐ Slightly ☐ Not very ☐

Ways of coping with disinhibition for family and carers

- Recognise that the problem is due to the brain injury, and try not to take it personally.

- Give direct feedback. If the brain-injured person behaves inappropriately, tell them so at the time.

- Be firm. It is important to be firm quite early on, and not to allow disinhibited behaviour to be rewarded. Set boundaries and limitations, and spell out clearly that certain behaviour is inappropriate. A consequence of not being firm is that the person's lack of control over their behaviour will increase if they don't have to try to control it.

- Distract the brain-injured person. Redirect their attention to more appropriate behaviour.

- Monitor and modify. Keep a record of what occurs immediately before the inappropriate behaviour. What are the triggers? An ABC chart is best: A = antecedents (what happens immediately before the behaviour); B = behaviour; C = consequences (what happens immediately after the behaviour). By identifying and changing the antecedents and consequences, many behaviours can be modified.

Behaviour management and strategies for more severe problems of disinhibition

- Devise a behavioural management system. This involves making sure that appropriate behaviour is rewarded, and that inappropriate behaviour has a negative consequence. Rewards might include ticks on a chart, tokens, or praise and attention. Inappropriate behaviour might involve withdrawal of attention or time out, where the person is given absolutely no attention at all for a limited period of five or ten minutes.

- Skills training. An improvement in skills leads to a reduction in challenging behaviour. Key skills, which can be learned, include anxiety management, assertiveness training and anger management.

- Reinforce other behaviour, or the absence of the target behaviour. For example, the brain-injured person gets a 5-minute chat for each 30-minute period free of the inappropriate behaviour. (This is called DRO, or differential reinforcement of other behaviour.)

Identify two practical strategies for trying to reduce disinhibited behaviour.

How relevant did you find this sheet? Very ☐ Slightly ☐ Not very ☐

Awareness skills quiz

1 How good do you think your awareness is of any difficulties you may have as a result of your brain injury?

Crystal clear ☐ Fairly good ☐ Mildly restricted ☐ Poor ☐

2 Sigmund Freud said that 'knowing thyself' was the purpose of therapy, and a goal to strive for. What part of the brain is usually connected with the ability to know yourself, have awareness, or reflect on yourself?

____

3 Tick which of these behaviours would fall into the category of showing good awareness, and cross those that probably show poor awareness:

- Recognising that you've made a mistake ☐
- Anticipating situations where you might have difficulty ☐
- Saying, 'I've always had a poor memory.' ☐
- Using a compensatory strategy such as a diary ☐
- Wanting to return to the same job as if nothing had happened ☐
- Recognising that your life is now different ☐
- Feeling sad for the losses in your life ☐
- Saying, 'I haven't got any problems, I'm exactly the same as before my injury.' ☐

4 Identify three ways that a person can improve their awareness:

____

____

____

5 Having poor awareness is related to which of the following?

(a) Poor outcome in return to work	YES ☐	NO ☐
(b) Fatiguability and tiredness	YES ☐	NO ☐
(c) Impaired interpersonal relationships	YES ☐	NO ☐

How relevant did you find this sheet? Very ☐ Slightly ☐ Not very ☐

EXERCISE 1

Personality/behaviour assessment

How difficult do you think you will find this exercise? Easy ☐ OK ☐ Quite difficult ☐ Very difficult ☐

Instruction

Look at the rating scale below, and circle the numbers that represent your personality now. Then in a different coloured pen, circle how you were before your injury.

Quick-tempered	1	2	3	4	5	6	7	8	9	10	Even-tempered
Reliant on others	1	2	3	4	5	6	7	8	9	10	I do things myself
Cold	1	2	3	4	5	6	7	8	9	10	Affectionate
Dislike company	1	2	3	4	5	6	7	8	9	10	Fond of company
Irritable	1	2	3	4	5	6	7	8	9	10	Easy-going
Unhappy	1	2	3	4	5	6	7	8	9	10	Happy
Excitable	1	2	3	4	5	6	7	8	9	10	Calm
Inactive	1	2	3	4	5	6	7	8	9	10	Energetic
Out of touch	1	2	3	4	5	6	7	8	9	10	Down to earth
Rash	1	2	3	4	5	6	7	8	9	10	Cautious
Listless	1	2	3	4	5	6	7	8	9	10	Enthusiastic
Childish	1	2	3	4	5	6	7	8	9	10	Mature
Insensitive	1	2	3	4	5	6	7	8	9	10	Sensitive
Forgetful	1	2	3	4	5	6	7	8	9	10	Mindful
Mean	1	2	3	4	5	6	7	8	9	10	Generous
Unreasonable	1	2	3	4	5	6	7	8	9	10	Reasonable
Lack of confidence	1	2	3	4	5	6	7	8	9	10	Self-confident
Emotional	1	2	3	4	5	6	7	8	9	10	Stable

Comment on and discuss the main changes.

How did you find this exercise? Easy ☐ OK ☐ Quite difficult ☐ Very difficult ☐

Social skills assessment

How difficult do you think you will find this exercise? Easy ☐ OK ☐ Quite difficult ☐ Very difficult ☐

Instruction

Fill in the questionnaire, identifying changes that you have noticed in the way you react in social situations, since your injury. Now get someone close to you to complete the questionnaire and fill in the independent scorer column. Discuss the scores.

Question	Self-score			Independent scorer		
	No change	Slight change	Some change	No change	Slight change	Some change
1 **Proximity:** When talking, I stand too close or too far away from people.						
2 **Eye contact:** I have poorer eye contact, look away more, or tend to stare more.						
3 **Facial expression:** My face is more, or less, expressive.						
4 **Speech volume:** My speech volume is either louder or quieter.						
5 **Speech speed:** I talk more quickly, or more slowly.						
6 **Speech intonation:** My voice is flatter and lacks intonation.						
7 **Word-finding:** In everyday conversation I sometimes cannot find the right word.						
8 **Going off the point, and getting to the point:** In everyday conversation I often stray off the point. Sometimes I miss the point. I might have difficulty expressing what I want to say precisely.						
9 **Taking turns in conversation:** I talk too much and do not allow the other person to have a turn.						
10 **Expressed emotion:** I express my emotions differently – either too much or too little. This might be getting angry more quickly, or less quickly, or feeling tearful and sad more or less quickly.						
11 **Self-disclosure:** I express myself more freely. I tell people what I think, and how I feel more readily.						
12 **Humour:** I sometimes make a joke or laugh at something inappropriately.						
13 **Recognising emotions in others:** I am less able to pick up and interpret how others are feeling.						
14 **Empathy:** I do not feel the same sensitivity to other people's feelings.						

Add any other changes in your social skills that you have noticed.

How did you find this exercise? Easy ☐ OK ☐ Quite difficult ☐ Very difficult ☐

Mood and emotions assessment

How difficult do you think you will find this exercise? Easy ☐ OK ☐ Quite difficult ☐ Very difficult ☐

Instruction

Fill in the questionnaire below, identifying changes that you have noticed in the way you react emotionally since your injury. Now get someone close to you to complete the questionnaire and fill in the independent scorer column. Discuss the scores.

Question	Self-score			Independent scorer		
	No change	Slight change	Some change	No change	Slight change	Some change
1 **Emotional lability:** I cry and/or laugh more easily than I used to.						
2 **Emotional flatness:** I have a reduced intensity of emotions, feeling emotionally rather flat – neither up nor down – blunted.						
3 **Lowered tolerance of frustration:** I have a tendency to anger more quickly, be more irritable, and snap over little things.						
4 **Suspicion:** I am more mistrusting of others, believing that others harbour malicious intent.						
5 **Anxiety:** I have more worry, fear, concerns about present and future.						
6 **Reduced motivation and drive:** I am more laid back, lacking previous drive and persistence, more apathetic.						
7 **Depression:** Low mood, pessimism, sadness, guilt, shame.						
8 **Reduced empathy:** Less able to feel sorry for others, and to 'put myself in their shoes'; more pre-occupied with myself.						
9 **Disinhibited:** I am more expressive – I can't keep feelings and thoughts to myself – they just come out more easily; sometimes I make socially inappropriate comments.						

Add any other emotional changes and discuss the most significant changes since your brain injury.

How did you find this exercise? Easy ☐ OK ☐ Quite difficult ☐ Very difficult ☐

Do I feel the same?

How difficult do you think you will find this exercise? Easy ☐ OK ☐ Quite difficult ☐ Very difficult ☐

Instruction

Read the following information, and provide some examples if it applies to you:

Lowered tolerance. Some people find that, following brain injury, they are less tolerant and lose their temper more quickly over little things. You might say, 'I've got a shorter fuse.' If this is the case, give a specific example of a situation where you have lost your temper more quickly:

➤

Emotional lability. Some people find that they get more emotional and tearful more quickly, often over small things. One person reported that they found themselves crying over sad items on the news, or a sentimental film. Usually the tears don't last long, and normal mood is re-established quickly. If you think this applies to you, give an example:

➤

Emotional flattening. Sometimes people find they do not experience the same depth and range of emotions – it's almost as if the emotions have been flattened off at an even level. One wife commented, 'when his mother died it did not seem to affect him as it would have done. All he said was, '"she had a good life and it comes to us all", and at the funeral he tended to laugh slightly inappropriately.' Do you feel things differently, or have others commented about how you might be different? Give an example:

➤

How did you find this exercise? Easy ☐ OK ☐ Quite difficult ☐ Very difficult ☐

My personality

How difficult do you think you will find this exercise? Easy ☐ OK ☐ Quite difficult ☐ Very difficult ☐

Instruction

1 Read through the list of adjectives, and circle the six that you think are most descriptive of you at present.

happy	insensitive	cautious	emotional
of value	unreasonable	stable	forgetful
independent	changeable	unhappy	withdrawn
energetic	even-tempered	helpless	stupid
quick-tempered	affectionate	anxious	inactive
rash	sociable	unattractive	irritable
childish	calm	lacking confidence	ambitious
self-centred	talkative	reliable	helpful
easy-going	enthusiastic	kind	mature

2 Identify personality characteristics that you think have changed since your accident:

I have become more ________ I have become less ________

I have become more ________ I have become less ________

I have become more ________ I have become less ________

3 Do people close to you think you have changed in any way? If so, in what ways do they say you have changed?

____

____

____

4 Ask your partner, or a close family member or friend, to answer the questions above and compare and discuss answers.

____

____

How did you find this exercise? Easy ☐ OK ☐ Quite difficult ☐ Very difficult ☐

Advertisement

How difficult do you think you will find this exercise? Easy ☐ OK ☐ Quite difficult ☐ Very difficult ☐

Instruction

Follow the headings below, and carefully select words that best describe yourself, in order to form an advertisement which will 'paint a picture of you'. The sheets will then be collected and redistributed within the group or family. People have to guess who the advertisement describes:

1 Appearance (three words only):

__________ __________ __________

2 Personality described as a: fruit __________

animal __________

musical instrument __________

3 Particular skills (three words only):

__________ __________ __________

4 My four biggest disabilities or problems are:

____

____

____

____

____

5 My biggest fear is (maximum of two words only):

__________ __________

How did you find this exercise? Easy ☐ OK ☐ Quite difficult ☐ Very difficult ☐

EXERCISE 7

Activities and personality

How difficult do you think you will find this exercise? Easy ☐ OK ☐ Quite difficult ☐ Very difficult ☐

Instruction

1 Make a list of all the activities you like doing. They can be activities you carry out alone or with others; activities you used to carry out, or activities you still carry out now; or activities you would like to carry out in the future. Fill in the table below, ticking the appropriate columns:

Activities you like doing	Before	Now	Future	Alone	With others

2 Once everyone in the group has compiled their lists, swap sheets with someone else. The other person then has to write down what these activities tell them about the personality of the person who compiled the list. Draw up a brief personality profile. Afterwards, discuss with the group.

Write down a personality profile based on the above list.

How did you find this exercise? Easy ☐ OK ☐ Quite difficult ☐ Very difficult ☐

Hobbies and leisure

How difficult do you think you will find this exercise? Easy ☐ OK ☐ Quite difficult ☐ Very difficult ☐

Instruction

1 What hobbies and leisure activities did you enjoy and spend time on before your injury?

➤	➤
➤	➤
➤	➤

2 Think of an activity that you continue to do, or you want to continue with, but you recognise that you have to do it differently – you have to compensate in some ways.

Activity	How can I carry out the activity differently

3 Identify two new activities that you could attempt, and give a reason why you think you might enjoy them. Be creative in your thinking.

New activity	Reasons why you think you might enjoy this activity
➤	➤
➤	➤

How did you find this exercise? Easy ☐ OK ☐ Quite difficult ☐ Very difficult ☐

Empathy

How difficult do you think you will find this exercise? Easy ☐ OK ☐ Quite difficult ☐ Very difficult ☐

Instruction

Lack of feelings of empathy, or the ability to 'put yourself in somebody else's shoes' and imagine how they feel, is a common problem after brain injury. This may be because you become preoccupied with your own problems, and/or due to direct cognitive impairment. Are you lacking in empathy? Complete the following questions to help you find out:

1 Name a person who is very close to you, and who has been affected by your accident:

____

2 What have been the two biggest changes or losses for that person since your injury?

➤ ______________________________

____

➤ ______________________________

____

3 Put yourself in their shoes. Describe how your injury and disability has affected them in different areas of their life:

➤ Social life

➤ Domestic duties

➤ Finance/work

➤ Emotional issues

4 What do you think have been the two most difficult changes in you for them to deal with?

➤ ______________________________

____

➤ ______________________________

____

How did you find this exercise? Easy ☐ OK ☐ Quite difficult ☐ Very difficult ☐

Motivation

How difficult do you think you will find this exercise? Easy ☐ OK ☐ Quite difficult ☐ Very difficult ☐

Instruction

People often find they feel different after any form of brain injury. They often say, 'I don't feel the same', or 'I don't have the same get up and go.' Sometimes people say they feel less motivated, and just don't want to do the things they did previously. Are you less motivated than you used to be? Complete the following questions to find out:

1 List five things that motivate you right now. These are things that energise you, or make you want to get up and do something.

2 What have you initiated in the last week? It could be something small or trivial, or something much larger.

3 Think of something that motivates you. Now make a plan involving that activity that you will carry out over the next few months.

How did you find this exercise? Easy ☐ OK ☐ Quite difficult ☐ Very difficult ☐

Disinhibition

How difficult do you think you will find this exercise? Easy ☐ OK ☐ Quite difficult ☐ Very difficult ☐

Instruction

Many people find they are more disinhibited after their brain injury – although you may not be aware of it. This means that you tend to have less control over your emotions, behaviour and actions – feelings and thoughts just slip out more easily. Are you more disinhibited? Complete the following to find out:

	Definitely	Sometimes	Not at all
1 I often find that I 'speak first.....think later'.			
2 I have greater difficulty controlling and concealing my feelings – they just spill out of me.			
3 I think that I am more impulsive, and often tend to do or say things without really thinking through the consequences.			
4 I sometimes make socially inappropriate comments or actions.			
5 I lose my temper more quickly – I just snap.			
6 Add any other examples.			

Give an example of a situation in which you think you have been disinhibited.

List the strategies you can use to help you cope with this problem. Discuss.

How did you find this exercise? Easy ☐ OK ☐ Quite difficult ☐ Very difficult ☐

Emotional tone – voices

How difficult do you think you will find this exercise? Easy ☐ OK ☐ Quite difficult ☐ Very difficult ☐

Instruction

Sometimes after a brain injury, people have problems expressing emotional tone in their voice or speech. Others have problems interpreting the emotional tone in other people's speech. One man who had a right-hemisphere stroke had great problems interpreting emotions in others. As he was a self-employed Information Technology Consultant, he often had to sit in meetings where people would say things, and he could never be sure whether they were angry, joking, or happy. Do you have problems with emotional tone? Complete the following questions to find out:

1 Have you noticed that your expressive speech has been affected by your injury in any way? If so, describe in what way.

____

____

____

2 Have you noticed that your ability to interpret others' emotions is altered in any way? If so, in what way?

____

____

____

3 If you are in a group, each person chooses a sentence from below and says it directly to one other member of the group in turn, using a negative (angry/critical) tone; a positive (kind/complimentary) tone, or a neutral tone. The rest of the group have to guess which tone is being used. If you are not in a group, try out the exercise on a friend or family member:

- 'Where did you get that tie (shirt, blouse, etc)?'
- 'When will dinner be ready?'
- 'When are you going?'
- 'When does this group end?'
- 'I had to come by bus today.'
- Make up your own sentence.

How did you find this exercise? Easy ☐ OK ☐ Quite difficult ☐ Very difficult ☐

Social blunders

How difficult do you think you will find this exercise? Easy ☐ OK ☐ Quite difficult ☐ Very difficult ☐

Instruction

Read the following true stories, and then try to identify the aspects of brain injury on the checklists at the bottom of the page that may have caused the social blunder.

Story 1: Mary

Mary was at a meeting with some friends from the local church, one of whom had unfortunately lost her son through a tragic accident. After a while, the topic of conversation turned to schools. Mary commented, 'I sent my son to Presentation College. If you had a son, where would you send him to school?' There was a moment's silence, and only then did Mary realise what she had said.

Story 2: Wayne

Wayne was a single, 25-year-old man who had sustained a brain injury five years ago and was keenly looking for a girlfriend. He had a part-time job in a supermarket, and had become quite friendly with one of the girls on the check-out. On one occasion he noticed her licking her lips when she was talking to him. Wayne misinterpreted this friendliness and her licking her lips as a 'come on'. He rather inappropriately bought a packet of condoms, and waving them in front of her asked her if she wanted to go out with him that night. The girl was very upset by this behaviour and burst into tears. She later complained to the manager and Wayne was sacked.

Rank in order, which of the factors below were most significant in causing each social blunder to happen.

	Story 1: Mary	**Story 2: Wayne**
1 Poor memory – difficulty remembering what has been said		
2 Poor sense of smell and taste		
3 Impulsiveness and disinhibition– tending to say and do the first thing that comes to mind		
4 Fatigue and tiredness – increasing tiredness leads to more likelihood of making a mistake		
5 Poor executive skills – problems holding more than one thing in mind at the same time, linking and integrating bits of information, thinking things through and reaching sound judgements		

Describe a situation where you have made a 'social blunder'; 'dropped a clanger', or 'got the wrong end of the stick'.

How did you find this exercise? Easy ☐ OK ☐ Quite difficult ☐ Very difficult ☐

Being flexible

How difficult do you think you will find this exercise? Easy ☐ OK ☐ Quite difficult ☐ Very difficult ☐

Instruction

After brain injury, people often become less flexible in their thinking and behaviour. Read the following humorous example, and then complete the tasks following it.

An armada of the US Navy was engaged in a naval exercise off the coast of Canada, when the following radio exchange was recorded:

➤**1** 'Please divert your course 15 degrees to the north to avoid danger of collision.'

➤**2** 'Recommend that you divert your course 15 degrees to the south to avoid danger of collision.'

➤**1** 'We repeat. Divert north now to avoid collision.'

➤**2** 'Strongly recommend you divert south soonest to avoid mishap.'

➤**1** 'This is the Captain of US Navy warship. I say again, divert your course with immediate effect.'

➤**2** 'Copy we say divert south now.'

➤**1** 'This is the USS Enterprise. We are an aircraft carrier of the US Navy. Divert your course NOW.'

➤**2** 'We are a Canadian lighthouse. Your call!'

We could all be more flexible at times. Think of an everyday situation where you recognise that you could have been more flexible.

➤

➤

Looking back on this situation, how might you have done things differently for a more positive outcome?

➤

How did you find this exercise? Easy ☐ OK ☐ Quite difficult ☐ Very difficult ☐

EXERCISE 15

Unusual symptoms

How difficult do you think you will find this exercise? Easy ☐ OK ☐ Quite difficult ☐ Very difficult ☐

Instruction

A brain injury can cause a large variety of different symptoms. The most obvious ones are changes in mobility, poor memory, concentration difficulties, fatigue, and lowered tolerance of stress and frustration. However, often people say they have noticed subtle, unusual changes, such as a lack of sensation in certain parts of their body, a lack of sense of time, difficulty with temperature, or even a lack of the ability to laugh or cry.

1 Write a list of unusual symptoms or changes in yourself that you have noticed since your brain injury. They may be physical, mental, or emotional.

2 Discuss as a group, or collect the completed sheets and hand them back to different members of the group, who then have to read out symptoms and guess who they belong to.

How did you find this exercise? Easy ☐ OK ☐ Quite difficult ☐ Very difficult ☐

Impulsivity

How difficult do you think you will find this exercise? Easy ☐ OK ☐ Quite difficult ☐ Very difficult ☐

Instruction

Being impulsive, or acting without thinking through the pros and cons of a situation, is a common problem after any brain injury. Read this example and then complete the rating chart that follows.

> Example: James
>
> One day, James bought £3,000 worth of shares in Marks & Spencer. He made the decision on impulse, as he had just read about the share price in the morning paper and happened to be walking past the bank. Before his brain injury, he would always have discussed such a major purchase with his wife, but on this occasion he made the decision without consulting her. Understandably, she was very angry.
>
> James likes shopping, but since his brain injury his judgement is somewhat suspect. On one occasion, he bought six bags of bananas because there was a special offer (three bags for the price of two), and he likes bananas. He did not bear in mind that they were going away on holiday, and most of the bananas would not be eaten and would rot.

Tick any of the following statements that might explain James' impulsiveness and put a cross alongside those that are not relevant.

1 He has difficulty holding in mind three or four 'bits' of information at the same time, and synthesising them – weighing them all up together and reaching a balanced decision.	
2 He suffers from fatigue, gets tired more easily, and needs more sleep.	
3 His brain is slower at processing information.	
4 The part of his brain that dampens down, checks, or inhibits impulses – the frontal lobes – is not working as well as it should. So he is generally rather disinhibited, saying and doing whatever comes into his mind without holding back.	

> *Describe a situation when you have been more impulsive since your injury.*

How did you find this exercise? Easy ☐ OK ☐ Quite difficult ☐ Very difficult ☐

EXERCISE 17

Changing roles

How difficult do you think you will find this exercise? Easy ☐ OK ☐ Quite difficult ☐ Very difficult ☐

Instruction

After a brain injury, many people cannot carry out the same roles as they did before. They and their family have to be flexible and change roles. Identify how roles might change by ticking the appropriate boxes on the chart that follows.

Roles	Could definitely do	Might be able to do	Would not be able to do
1 Shopping – buys the majority of family shopping			
2 Cooking – the majority of family weekday evening meals			
3 Pays bills – organises finances			
4 Breadwinner – primary money earner			
5 DIY – house maintenance			
6 Chauffeur – driving children to their activities			
7 Househusband – tidies up and cleans the house			
8 Helping children with homework			
9 Taking children to school and picking up			
10 Disciplinarian – setting and enforcing rules with children			
11 Playing games – and organising activities with children			
12 Responsible for walking the dog once a day			

Think about how your roles have changed since your brain injury, and fill in the boxes below. Discuss

Roles lost ➤ ➤	➤ ➤ ➤
New roles ➤ ➤	➤ ➤ ➤
Roles that I could take on ➤ ➤	➤ ➤ ➤

How did you find this exercise? Easy ☐ OK ☐ Quite difficult ☐ Very difficult ☐

Sinking in

How difficult do you think you will find this exercise? Easy ☐ OK ☐ Quite difficult ☐ Very difficult ☐

Instruction

The idea of this exercise is to trace your moods back over time since your injury. Have there been any major mood fluctuations, and were they linked to particular events? Look at the example and then try to fill in your own mood graphs and discuss.

Time/life events	Injury / Leaving hospital / At home alone / Return to work / Failing at work
High **Mood fluctuations** Low	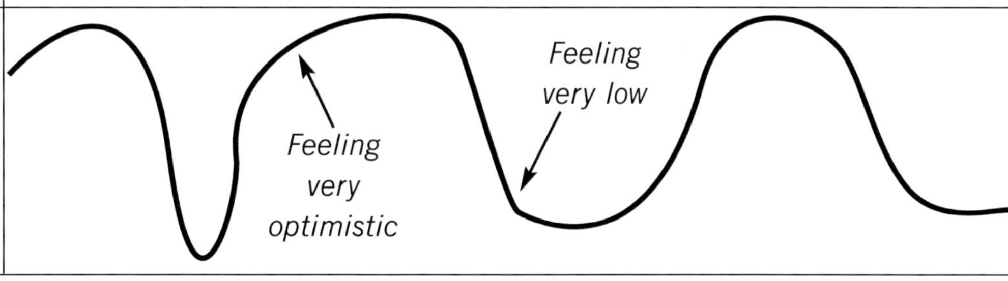

Time/life events	Injury
High **Mood fluctuations** Low	

Time/life events	
High **Mood fluctuations** Low	

How did you find this exercise? Easy ☐ OK ☐ Quite difficult ☐ Very difficult ☐

Who am I?

How difficult do you think you will find this exercise? Easy ☐ OK ☐ Quite difficult ☐ Very difficult ☐

Instruction

'I wonder if I've changed in the night … Let me think: was I the same when I got up this morning? … But if I'm not the same, the next question is, who am I? That's the great puzzle.'

Lewis Carroll: *Alice's Adventures in Wonderland*

Like Alice, many people who survive a brain injury feel changed. The cognitive skills involved in thinking and remembering are impaired; emotions and feelings may be experienced differently; physical changes occur – all of which creates a distorted picture of reality. Many people have difficulty seeing themselves from other people's points of view. In order to accept what has happened and move on in your life, it helps to develop an awareness of your 'new self'.

Write a description of yourself as if you were talking about a friend – for example, Tony Brown. Be sure to write it in the third person. For example, start by saying, 'Tony Brown is…….'. Start with what the person (you) looks like, as if you were asked to pick them out in a crowd. Then go into more detail about their personality, and what you think about them.

Write here:

How did you find this exercise? Easy ☐ OK ☐ Quite difficult ☐ Very difficult ☐

My coat of arms

How difficult do you think you will find this exercise? Easy ☐ OK ☐ Quite difficult ☐ Very difficult ☐

Instruction

In the Middle Ages, in the times of heraldry and knights in shining armour, people used to have coats of arms, bearing symbols, mottos and epitaphs. Design your own coat of arms, including your thoughts about yourself.

My biggest success of the year	My biggest failure of the year
Hope for next year	Hope for 10 years from now
Motto	Epitaph

How did you find this exercise? Easy ☐ OK ☐ Quite difficult ☐ Very difficult ☐

Are you joking?

How difficult do you think you will find this exercise? Easy ☐ OK ☐ Quite difficult ☐ Very difficult ☐

Instruction

It sometimes happens that after a brain injury, people's sense of humour alters. Read the following jokes, and identify the best possible punchline of the three on offer at the bottom:

1 A kangaroo walks into a bar and asks for a pint of beer. The barman, astonished, gives the kangaroo his drink. 'How much?' asks the animal. The barman recovers his composure and decides to see if the kangaroo is really as clever as he seems. Winking knowingly at the other customers at the bar, he says, 'Twenty-five pounds.' The kangaroo duly pays this, and the barman, reassured of the continuing superiority of his own species, relaxes and says: 'Don't get many kangaroos in here.'

- (i) The kangaroo pulls out a gun and shoots the barman.
- (ii) The man on the next stool admits that he is a ventriloquist who has trained the kangaroo to drink beer.
- (ii) 'I'm not surprised,' replies the kangaroo, 'with beer at that price.'

2 I had toothache the other day and went to the dentist. He said, 'lie back and say "Aahh."' I said, 'Why?' He said:

- (i) 'Because I want to see your tonsils.'
- (ii) 'Because my dog died yesterday.'
- (iii) 'Because I want to see if you can sing.'

Has your sense of humour changed at all since your injury, and if so, in what way? For example, do you laugh more, or less, or at the same things?

How did you find this exercise? Easy ☐ OK ☐ Quite difficult ☐ Very difficult ☐

EXERCISE 22

'Getting the wrong end of the stick'

How difficult do you think you will find this exercise? Easy ☐ OK ☐ Quite difficult ☐ Very difficult ☐

Instruction

The world we live in is full of subtle cues or 'bits of information' that our brains need to process and respond to. Sometimes after a head injury, people might misinterpret subtle social cues and reach the wrong conclusions.

Katie's story

Sometimes I just get the wrong end of the stick – reach wrong conclusions in social situations. The worst incident occurred when I texted my old boss from university about a sailing event for the Naval Reserves at Bristol University. In my message, I put something like BUSC – meaning Bristol University Sailing Club. He texted back saying 'Brighton or Bristol for a long weekend.' I thought he was propositioning me, so I responded by writing 'You are a married man with kids. I am not interested.' He responded straight away saying, 'I think you've got your wires crossed. I was just enquiring whether the course was on at Bristol or Brighton.' I felt such an idiot – so embarrassed. It's like sometimes I see two and two and make five.

Rank in order which of these cognitive deficits may have been most to least responsible for Katie's error.

1 Poor memory – I forget vital bits of information.	
2 Poor executive skills – difficulty processing and synthesising multiple subtle pieces of information and reaching a sound judgement.	
3 Word-finding difficulties – sometimes the wrong words come out.	

Think of a social situation where you have 'misread the situation', or 'jumped to the wrong conclusion' and ended up feeling embarrassed.

Have you ever felt slightly 'paranoid' – misinterpreted 'cues' and come to the conclusion, based on fear, that something bad was going to happen? Give an example.

How did you find this exercise? Easy ☐ OK ☐ Quite difficult ☐ Very difficult ☐

How good is my awareness?

How difficult do you think you will find this exercise? Easy ☐ OK ☐ Quite difficult ☐ Very difficult ☐

Instruction

Rate your skills on the following charts, and then discuss the results.

1	No problem	Mild problem	Moderate problem	Severe problem
a My short-term memory and attention is ...				
b My ability to plan and organise – my executive skills are ...				
c My emotional stability (temper control and moodiness) is ...				

2	Describe two situations
a My short-term memory and attention is most likely to let me down in the following situations.	➤ ➤
b My ability to plan, organise and do more than one thing at a time (executive skills), is likely to let me down in the following situations:	➤ ➤
c I am most likely to lose my temper in the following situations. These are the triggers that make me angry:	➤ ➤

3	Strategies
a What strategies do you use to improve your memory?	
b What strategies do you use to improve your executive skills (planning, organising and multitasking ability)?	
c What strategies do you use to control your short temper, or another emotional difficulty that you have noticed?	

How did you find this exercise? Easy ☐ OK ☐ Quite difficult ☐ Very difficult ☐

Ways of improving awareness

How difficult do you think you will find this exercise? Easy ☐ OK ☐ Quite difficult ☐ Very difficult ☐

Instruction

It takes time for people with a brain injury to become fully aware of all their difficulties. There is usually a gradual dawning, or realisation. Although 'time' is a great healer and improver of insight, there are ways of speeding up that process. Tick which of the following ways of improving insight you use or have used:

		Whether used
1	Read books, leaflets and printed information about brain injury.	
2	Ask for, and listen to, feedback from friends and family about how I am now.	
3	Attend a group where I meet others with similar difficulties – learn from them.	
4	See myself on video.	
5	Make mistakes and fail, but learn from those mistakes and failures.	
6	Fill in questionnaires and checklists to help identify problems.	
7	Ask to be sent medical letters and reports, and look at scans and other medical information.	
8	Have psychometric tests to assess memory, concentration and executive skills, and get feedback.	
9	Carry out rehabilitation exercises and games deliberately intended to highlight a problem.	
10	Engage in 'adjustment counselling' from a therapist who specialises in brain injury.	

List any other ways that have helped improve your insight.

➤

➤

➤

Which ways of improving insight have been most important to you personally? Choose your top three methods.

➤

➤

➤

How did you find this exercise? Easy ☐ OK ☐ Quite difficult ☐ Very difficult ☐

My profile

How difficult do you think you will find this exercise? Easy ☐ OK ☐ Quite difficult ☐ Very difficult ☐

Instruction

Fill in the questionnaire below, marking the column on the right-hand side with a tick, to signify how you view yourself compared with the average population of people your age. Do you see yourself as being above or below average on the particular measures?

	Very low range	Low average	Average range	High average	Superior range
Physical					
1 **Physical:** dexterity, movement, mobility, balance, strength					
2 **Sensory:** hearing, vision, taste, smell, touch					
3 **Fatigue:** tiredness, stamina, ability to continue without sleep					
Cognitive					
4 **Memory:** short-term remembering, new learning					
5 **Thinking:** attention, concentration, speed of processing					
6 **Executive functioning:** planning, organising, multitasking					
7 **Language:** word-finding, fluency, understanding complexity					
Temperamental					
8 **Tolerance of frustration:** ability to cope with frustration and stress					
9 **Moodiness fluctuations:** changeability, variability in mood					
10 **Emotional flatness:** limited range of emotions, little variation					
11 **Disinhibition:** expressive, talkative, emotions that just slip out					
12 **Motivation and drive:** initiative, spark, 'get up and go', desire, ability and ambition					

After marking out how you are now, try to mark where you would have been before your injury. Discuss the gap.

How did you find this exercise? Easy ☐ OK ☐ Quite difficult ☐ Very difficult ☐

PART III

Adjustment Skills

INFORMATION SHEETS

ADJUSTMENT SKILLS EXERCISES

Adjustment skills questionnaire

Name ______________________________ Date ____________________

This questionnaire assesses your adjustment to the consequences of your brain injury. Read each of the statements, and mark the box that best describes your beliefs at present. It might be helpful to ask someone who knows you well to complete the questionnaire and fill in the independent scorer column. Compare the two columns.

Scoring Agree = 2 Partially agree = 1 Disagree = 0

Question	**Score**					
	Self-score			Independent scorer		
	Agree	Partially agree	Disagree	Agree	Partially agree	Disagree
1 The injury was a turning point in my life.						
2 I can talk openly to people about my injury and the difficulties that I have had since then.						
3 I generally feel comfortable with myself and my life.						
4 I no longer keep comparing myself with how I used to be before the injury.						
5 I recognise my limitations now – things I cannot do.						
6 I can recognise that there have been some positive consequences of my injury.						
7 How I manage in the future depends on me, and not on what others do for me.						
8 I do not feel particularly anxious or depressed.						
9 I have a second chance, as I could have died; the future is now a new chapter in my life.						
10 I can still live a satisfying life, even though I might have some hidden disabilities as a result of my brain injury.						
TOTAL SCORE						

INTERPRETATION

Self-score

0–10: This suggests that the difficult process of adjustment might still be ongoing.

Discrepancy between self-score and independent score

5–20: This suggests that there is a difference between how you and others feel that you have adjusted.

How relevant did you find this sheet? Very ☐ Slightly ☐ Not very ☐

What is adjustment?

Emotional adjustment to disability resulting from brain injury is about accepting that life is now different. It can be likened to the process of bereavement, in which there is a coming to terms with the loss of a loved one. The word bereavement actually means 'to be robbed of something'.
The process involves both emotionally processing and accepting the loss, and then reorganising your thinking and lifestyle to accommodate that loss.

Adjustment to brain injury is particularly difficult, and may take years because of a number of factors:

- It is often a hidden loss or hidden disability – you usually can't see it. If you had a big plaster on your head, or you were missing a leg, it would be easier. Often other people do not recognise that you have problems.
- Spontaneous recovery continues for the first few years, and then tends to plateau off. You may think, 'I'm going to get better', and will not want to accept that recovery will be only partial.
- Awareness occurs gradually, as cognitive skills improve. You were probably not aware of what happened in the accident. You may have been unconscious, and will have taken time to catch up on this information.
- It is very difficult to be objective about yourself – other people see things about you that you do not. Often, it takes exposure to practical situations where you do not perform as well, to help you recognise that your abilities might be limited.
- The part of the brain that deals with self-awareness and insight – the frontal lobe – is usually the very part that is damaged in a brain injury.

There are a number of stages in bereavement:

- **Shock.** The reality of the loss takes time to sink in, and people react in different ways – denial, hysteria, disbelief, or confusion.
- **Protest.** At this stage, strong and powerful feelings occur, such as anger, guilt, sadness, fear, yearning, and searching as you struggle between the fantasy of denying, and the reality of accepting, what has happened.
- **Disorganisation.** This is the stage when the reality of the loss is only too real, and you may feel despair and depression.
- **Reorganisation.** You begin to rebuild your life, acquiring more balance, and being able to remember happier times again.

Signs of adjustment:

- Have you accepted that things will never quite be the same? Life has changed, and you are now developing fresh horizons and goals.
- Can you identify exactly what your problems are? Can you accurately list your top five problems as a result of your brain injury?

What is adjustment?

- Do you use strategies for compensating? These can vary from using a diary or notebook to cutting down on activities that are too demanding.
- Can you talk about it? Emotional adjustment implies that the emotion associated with the trauma or loss is no longer so devastating as to be deeply upsetting. A good test of this is whether you can talk to others about your losses in an open and honest way.
- Have you integrated your disability into your identity, and accepted your limitations?
- Have you recreated a new, balanced lifestyle in terms of different activities at work, home and leisure? This means not constantly striving to do things that are ultimately going to be disappointing and frustrating.

Adjustment ultimately means letting go of the old, and embracing the new. This may mean letting go of old habits, goals, ideas, aspirations and dreams, accepting your new limitations and looking towards new horizons.

1 What factors make adjustment to brain injury potentially more difficult than adjustment to a purely physical disability?

2 What stages are usually involved in bereavement? Which stage do you think you are most closely involved in?

3 Identify three signs that might indicate a positive adjustment.

How relevant did you find this sheet? Very ☐ Slightly ☐ Not very ☐

Goal-planning after brain injury

Human beings are goal-directed creatures, constantly striving for meaning, significance and purpose. We all need something to work towards – something to achieve. A lack of goals, unrealistic goals, or having too many goals, can result in stress.

Research suggests that people who are the most successful tend to be goal planners. Setting and working towards goals increases motivation and releases stores of energy. In studies of survivors of stressful environments, such as concentration camps, the best equipped to survive were those who created goals to work towards.

People often do not set goals, because they do not know how to; they do not realise the importance of goal-planning; or they have a deep-seated fear of failure. Once a goal is set and written down, the effect is usually to increase commitment and motivation.

Steps in goal-planning

- **Brainstorm.** Decide what you really want out of life. Identify and write down goals for home, work, leisure and personal development.
- **Re-examine.** Once you have generated this list, go back and look at it closely identifying which goals are realistic, and which might be unobtainable.
- **Rewrite the goals in terms of an outcome.** Write out your modified goal in clear, specific language, in terms of an actual outcome. For example, 'By next Christmas I will have walked two miles round a running track.'
- **Write out an action plan.** Break your goal into small steps that are needed to achieve it. They should be very specific, not vague.
- **Identify obstacles.** These are the things that will get in the way of you achieving your goals.
- **Build in rewards, and visualise the end result.** Have a clear mental picture of what you want to achieve to increase motivation.

1 Identify three reasons why goal-planning is important.
2 Write out one specific goal, with an action plan, or four or five steps, and identify potential obstacles.

How relevant did you find this sheet? Very ☐ Slightly ☐ Not very ☐

Anger management

A lowered tolerance to frustration, and a tendency to get angry more quickly, are very common results of any form of brain injury, particularly when the frontal lobe of the brain is damaged. People talk of being more disinhibited, or being unable to control their emotional impulses.

Humans ideally develop from being a screaming baby with no emotional control, through childhood and adolescence to being an adult who can think before expressing emotions: our brains mature. This means that our brain cells are wiring together to form neural pathways, or structures that help us to control behaviour and inhibit primitive impulses. After brain injury, these neural pathways are shaken up and become damaged.

Alongside this problem of disinhibition, involving the damaged frontal lobes, the person with a brain injury is under enormous stresses in everyday life. It is extremely frustrating to keep forgetting things; to make careless errors, to be less quick-witted, or to keep getting headaches. This stress creates anger.

Ways of managing anger after brain injury

Anticipate the triggers. Identify which situations are going to 'wind you up', by keeping a record of when and where you lose your temper. It might be in a very demanding situation, when you make silly mistakes, or when people speak to you in a particular way. Everyone has particular triggers to which they are most sensitive. Then do something to alter these triggers, to avoid them, or to find a way around them.

Identify and express the feelings beneath the anger. Underneath anger there is often hurt, fear, rejection, or a feeling of being threatened, or ignored. Try to express this emotion rather than the anger. One parent said to his daughter, who was busily chatting to her mother, 'When you two get talking like that, I feel ignored and rejected, and even more useless than normal. Remember that I am still here.' It is a positive experience to express negative feelings in a clear, non-blaming way, and it reduces stress.

Identify and challenge your rigid 'should,' 'must' and 'ought' beliefs. The core beliefs behind anger are usually those kinds of internal mental commands that involve the words 'should,' 'must' and 'ought.' If we could delete the word 'should' from our internal vocabulary, we would all be happier people. Challenge why things 'should' be so, and replace the word 'should' with 'it would be nice if…' After brain injury, thinking often becomes more rigid and less flexible, and words such as 'should' get used more readily.

Anger management

Visualise and imagine yourself in situations of high stress. Visualise coping differently in situations where you might be prone to lose your temper – close your eyes and imagine exactly what you would do.

Get into a regular routine that is not too demanding. The more regular the routine the better.

Talk to people about your difficulties – particularly if they know about brain injury.

Manage your stress by pacing yourself, and maintain a balance in your life. If you are tired, take rest or sleep. Are you doing enough things that you enjoy?

Rearrange your timetable. For example, if you find it difficult when your teenage children invite their friends around to the house, make sure that it is at a time when you can either go out or have something relaxing to do.

Prepare positive self-statements. Identify key thoughts you can write down and repeat to yourself in times of high provocation. One man identified three words beginning with 'c' which he repeated to himself under his breath when he felt himself losing his temper. These were:

- ➤ Children – The children are just playing, they are not trying to wind me up.
- ➤ Challenge – Treat this as a challenge.
- ➤ Calm – Stay calm, try to relax.

Develop a calming routine. Go through it when you are feeling provoked:

- ➤ Relax your muscles, drop your shoulders, loosen your hands, and relax your jaw.
- ➤ Take two to three deep breaths from your stomach and not your chest.
- ➤ Count to 10.
- ➤ Distract yourself.

Leave the situation. Walk away if you feel you are losing it, remove yourself from the situation. Identify a safe place to go.

> **1** Why do people who have had a brain injury lose their temper more quickly?
> **2** Identify two 'triggers' that you recognise cause you to feel angry.
> **3** Identify at least three strategies that you could use to try to manage your temper.

How relevant did you find this sheet? Very ☐ Slightly ☐ Not very ☐

Depression

Depression can often follow a period of challenging rehabilitation, and the accompanying frustration and growing awareness that progress is gradual. This often coincides with reduced progress or gains, the realisation of all the losses, improved awareness and an acknowledgement that life will never be the same again.

Depression can be viewed as an inevitable stage of adjustment following brain injury – almost a stage that people have to go through to fully adjust. Going through a period of depression can be viewed as a sign of progress and moving forward.

Practical ways of coping with depression

1 Talk about how you feel to friends, family, or a counsellor – don't bottle it up.

2 Learn more about your new disability and its complexities – read about it.

3 View your situation as a road that you are on: a journey full of obstacles and challenges. View problems as challenges.

4 Try not to keep comparing life with how it was before the injury. Instead, compare life with how it was immediately after.

5 Monitor your progress – keep a diary.

6 Join a brain injury support group, such as Headway – see how others cope.

7 Work towards just enjoying the pleasure of the moment, rather than the pleasure of achievements.

8 Set some goals – break down large tasks into small activities.

9 Lower your expectations.

10 Write down your negative thoughts and challenge them.

11 Get professional help if you feel really desperate.

> 1 Why is depression sometimes a sign of progress after brain injury?
> 2 Identify four positive ways of coping that you might implement if depressed.

How relevant did you find this sheet? Very ☐ Slightly ☐ Not very ☐

Dealing with fatigue

The disabling effects of fatigue can be extremely limiting in themselves. However, fatigue has a secondary negative effect on memory and concentration skills, tolerance and irritability levels, and physical symptoms such as headaches. A vicious circle is often formed, in which mental effort leads to fatigue, which leads to impaired mental skills and irritation, which leads to more fatigue. Approximately 70 per cent of people with a brain injury suffer from fatigue.

Mental effort such as concentration on office work is, for most people, a great trigger of fatigue, often more so than physical effort. People often describe it as being 'like a curtain coming down', or just suddenly 'running out of petrol'.

Fatigue is thought to be due to a number of causes. For example, after a brain injury your brain wants more sleep to be able to recover, and therefore sends the message: 'Close down, let's rest.' Also, it is thought that damage to the small nucleus in the middle of the brain, called the hypothalamus, affects arousal levels, sleep patterns and wakefulness.

Ways of coping with fatigue

1. **Recognise the early warning signs**, and do not keep pushing yourself. Take a rest. If you keep pushing yourself, serious fatigue will set in, and you will be wiped out for the whole day. Avoid the boom and bust cycle whereby you alternate between feeling fine and then exhausted.

2. **Pace yourself.** This means planning your days so that you do not overdo it. Build in rests – do not feel bad about having a sleep in the afternoon. Get into a regular routine that suits you. As you feel more able, gradually build up your routine.

3. **Say 'No' to the excessive demands of others**, and delegate tasks. Be open about your problem, and tell people that you suffer from fatigue.

4. **Do your most demanding activity in the morning**, when you have most mental energy.

5. **Eating a meal** can often boost energy levels.

1. What is the most common trigger to fatigue after brain injury?
2. Identify three strategies that you could adopt to cope with fatigue.
3. Identify any other ways of coping with fatigue.

How relevant did you find this sheet? Very ☐ Slightly ☐ Not very ☐

Assertiveness

Assertiveness describes a pattern of behaviour whereby you express your feelings and thoughts openly and honestly, and in a manner that does not violate the rights of other people. Assertiveness means standing up for yourself, being able to ask for what you want. It also means being able to say 'no' to the requests of others. By not standing up for yourself, your self-esteem goes down, and you are likely to feel under more stress.

Key assertiveness skills after brain injury

➤ **Saying no.** This is a vital self-protective skill after a brain injury, since you have got to reduce demands from others. When you say no, you are refusing a request, not rejecting a person – it is important to recognise that these things are quite different. After a brain injury, you simply cannot do as much. It may be difficult to say no, because a part of you does not want to accept that things have changed.

➤ **Self-disclosure.** This is an important skill, and involves disclosing how you are feeling, and how you would like people to treat you. For example, one man at work would say to his colleagues, 'I can't do more than one thing at a time since my accident.' Another example was a man at work who told his colleagues about his brain injury, and told them that from now on he wanted to work with his office door shut so that he was not continually interrupted. You have got to educate other people because they will not know much about brain injury.

➤ **Delegation.** Delegation means getting things done, or achieving goals through the efforts of other people. It is a major skill, whether in business or at home. Now you cannot do as much as you used to do, you need to be able to delegate. The benefits of delegation are that it gives you more time, increases your productivity, helps others take responsibility, and forces you to plan and organise. Some fears and obstacles to delegation include feeling guilty, feeling like a failure; fear of letting go, and fear of other people being more successful.

1 Identify one particular situation that you need either to say 'no' to, or to delegate.
2 What simple statement could you say to people to let them know that you have a problem, and to indicate that you do not want to take on a task straight away?

How relevant did you find this sheet? Very ☐ Slightly ☐ Not very ☐

Time management after brain injury

Time is the most scarce and valuable resource that we have in our lives. If we can manage our time, we can manage our life.

Know your goals in life. Identify what is important in your life. These goals that you are working towards are the map by which you give direction to your life.

Rank your priorities. Rank activities in terms of what is important to you, and what is less important. Ask: 'How important is this to me?'

Plan and write it down. Minutes spent in planning will be saved many times over. Using a diary, a calendar, or a 'to do' list, try to stand back. When you are feeling listless, make a list!

Delegate tasks. What can you hand over to other people to do? Delegation is a key way of managing your time.

Work out a system. Muddle makes unnecessary work, wastes time and creates frustration. Spend time organising your environment so 'there is a place for everything and everything is in its place.'

Learn to say no. If you cannot turn off the tap of demands and requests from others, you simply have no control over your life.

One thing at a time. We may have many things to do, but we cannot do them all at the same time. It is important to concentrate on particular tasks.

Leave slack in your timetable. Never fill up your timetable completely; always allow a little slack or leeway.

Overcome perfectionism. If you have to get everything absolutely right, you will find it difficult. Dare to be average sometimes.

Keep a balance. Spend time in a balance between work, home, leisure, physical activity and mental activity. Plan natural breaks during the day.

1 Identify three key time management skills that you could, or do use.
2 Which of the above areas of time management are you poor at?

How relevant did you find this sheet? Very ☐ Slightly ☐ Not very ☐

Adjustment skills quiz

1 How well do you think you have adjusted to life after your brain injury?

Reasonably well ☐ Fairly well ☐ Not well ☐ Poorly ☐

2 There is usually a sequence of emotional stages that people pass through after brain injury. Arrange the following emotions in what you would consider to be the most common order. Number the emotions from 1 to 6.

Depression	Anger	Adjustment	Shock	Denial	Acceptance
☐	☐	☐	☐	☐	☐

3 Rate which of these statements is the best, and which is the worst, description of adjustment to life after brain injury. Number them from 1 to 4.

Accepting that life has changed and you've got to get on with it.	
Recognising your limitations, and lowering your expectations of yourself.	
Continually striving to get back to how things were.	
Seeing your life now as a 'second chance' or 'new chapter'.	

4 Write a sentence that would be a definition of a good adjustment after brain injury:

____

____

5 Tick which of these behaviours would fall into the category of showing good adjustment, and cross those that probably show poor awareness:

- ➤ Talking openly about your brain injury and subsequent difficulties ☐
- ➤ Being comfortable with yourself ☐
- ➤ Comparing your present abilities and lifestyle with your pre-injury abilities and lifestyle ☐
- ➤ Having realistic goals and plans for the future ☐
- ➤ Accepting that your injury was a life-changing moment ☐
- ➤ Talking about 'getting back to normal' ☐
- ➤ Comparing yourself with others ☐
- ➤ Having the same expectations for yourself as you've always had ☐

6 Identify one way that a person can improve their adjustment:

____

How relevant did you find this sheet? Very ☐ Slightly ☐ Not very ☐

EXERCISE 1

The tree of life

How difficult do you think you will find this exercise? Easy ☐ OK ☐ Quite difficult ☐ Very difficult ☐

Instruction

The picture below represents a number of different images associated with feelings about life:

- Pick out the person who most closely represents how you feel about your life at the moment. Discuss as a group.
- Pick out a person you could most identify with from your past.

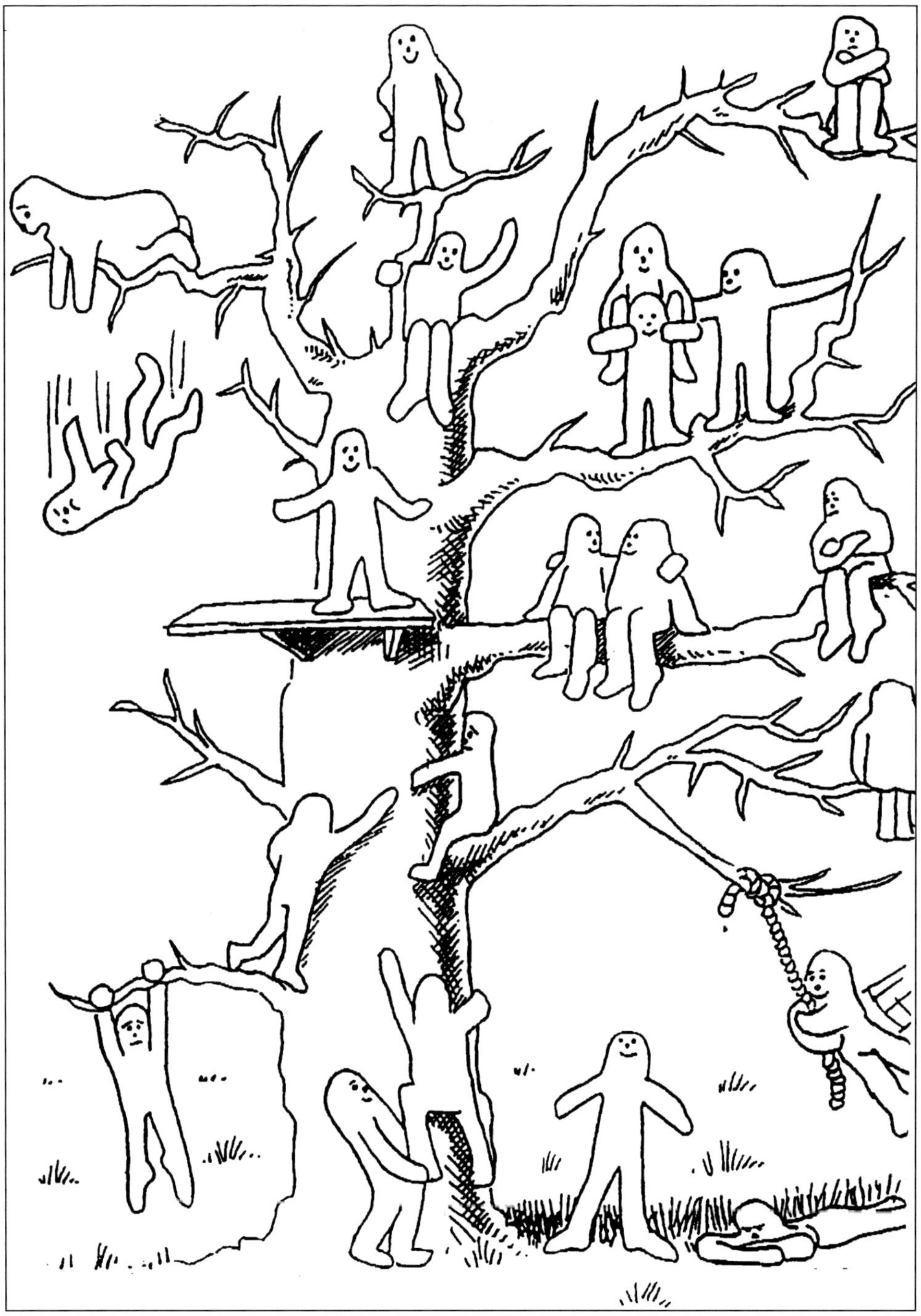

Reproduced with permission. Pip Wilson, Romford YMCA

How did you find this exercise? Easy ☐ OK ☐ Quite difficult ☐ Very difficult ☐

Why me?

How difficult do you think you will find this exercise? Easy ☐ OK ☐ Quite difficult ☐ Very difficult ☐

Instruction

It is common after any kind of trauma to ask ourselves the question, 'Why me?' This exercise tries to explore this issue.

1 How often do you ruminate on the thought: 'Why did it happen to me?'

More than once a day? ☐ Daily? ☐ Occasionally? ☐ Rarely? ☐ Never? ☐

2 Answer the question, 'Why did it have to happen to me?' in as many different ways as you can. Brainstorm: be as creative as you can. Here are a few initial ideas:

1 It was fate, God's will.
2 It was just bad luck.
3 It was punishment for my previous sins.
4 It was my fault… my carelessness.
5 It is better that it happened to me at my age than when I was younger, or to somebody else.

3 Consider the options above, and write down the one most believable answer to the question 'Why me?'

➤

4 Discuss as a group your answers to this question. Examine, in particular, people's tendency to either blame somebody or something else when something bad happens, or to blame themselves.

How did you find this exercise? Easy ☐ OK ☐ Quite difficult ☐ Very difficult ☐

Helpful and unhelpful approaches

How difficult do you think you will find this exercise? Easy ☐ OK ☐ Quite difficult ☐ Very difficult ☐

Instruction

The table below identifies a number of common problems after a brain injury, followed by a number of helpful or unhelpful ways for others to approach these problems. Look at the examples and then add some of your own helpful and unhelpful suggested approaches in the spaces provided.

Common Problems	**Unhelpful approach**	**Helpful approach**
Attention – poor – easily distracted	Two people talking at same time. ➤	One talker – reduce background noise ➤
Memory – forgetful	Giving too much information in one go ➤	Write it down. Repeat things ➤
Executive ability – problems multi-tasking.	Given several tasks to do at the same time ➤	One thing at a time. ➤
Insight and Awareness – not being fully aware of own problems.	Going along with denying the problem. ➤	Point out the problem gently. ➤
Lower tolerance of frustration – angers easily.	Being given instruction in a stern demanding tone of voice. ➤	Speak softly but firmly. ➤
Emotional Lability – cries or laughs more easily	Making too much fuss – 'oh poor old you'. ➤	Show awareness and then provide distraction. ➤
Emotionally flat – apathetic, little motivation	Being left to get on with it. ➤	Provide structure, prompts and incentives. ➤
Add your own.	➤	➤

How did you find this exercise? Easy ☐ OK ☐ Quite difficult ☐ Very difficult ☐

Over- and under-protectiveness

How difficult do you think you will find this exercise? Easy ☐ OK ☐ Quite difficult ☐ Very difficult ☐

Instruction

It is often difficult for family and carers to judge how to respond to someone with a brain injury. There is a fine line between being over-protective and doing too much, and being under-protective and doing too little.

1 Identify which of these examples is more likely to be over-protective, and which might be under-protective.

A John has a poor memory, and his mother doesn't like him going out on his own in case he gets lost. He is in his early twenties, and has lived at his family home all of his life.	
B Mrs Riley, aged 45, has always provided for her large family – the older children are now in their late teens and early twenties, but still live at home. She cooks, shops and cleans, and has a part-time job. Since her head injury, she suffers from fatigue and struggles to manage her huge workload. Her children and husband have never helped much, and assume that Mum will always cope.	

2 Think of an example when someone close to you has been over-protective, and done something for you that you didn't want them to do. Describe that situation.

____

____

____

3 Think of an example when someone close to you has been under-protective, and has allowed you do something that you couldn't manage. Describe that situation.

____

____

____

4 Take one of the above examples, and try to imagine how the other person might be feeling. What could you say to alter the situation?

____

____

How did you find this exercise? Easy ☐ OK ☐ Quite difficult ☐ Very difficult ☐

EXERCISE 5

'Oh, you do look well!'

How difficult do you think you will find this exercise? Easy ☐ OK ☐ Quite difficult ☐ Very difficult ☐

Instruction

1 The following statements are responses you might make to somebody who you know quite well who says 'You look well'. You do not feel well. Rank the statements in order of which you are most likely to say. Then discuss as a group.

1 I may look well, but I've still got lots of problems – if you've got a couple of hours I'll tell you about them.	
2 Push off, you creep.	
3 That's the last thing in the world I want somebody to say to me – I feel awful.	
4 You don't understand.	
5 I'm improving, and may look well, but under the bonnet there are a few problems.	
6 Yes, I'm fine thanks.	

2 Write down, in note form, the comments you would make to somebody who was asking how you are, and who genuinely wanted to know and had time to listen. What would you say? One person came up with the phrase, 'I look too disabled to be classed as normal, and too normal to be classed as disabled.'

How did you find this exercise? Easy ☐ OK ☐ Quite difficult ☐ Very difficult ☐

EXERCISE 6

Life map

How difficult do you think you will find this exercise? Easy ☐ OK ☐ Quite difficult ☐ Very difficult ☐

Instruction

Plot out a map, or pathway of your life. Use pictures or words to mark in significant events or turning points, such as births, marriages, deaths, moves and jobs. Start at your birth; work your way through to your injury, and then predict your future on the road ahead.

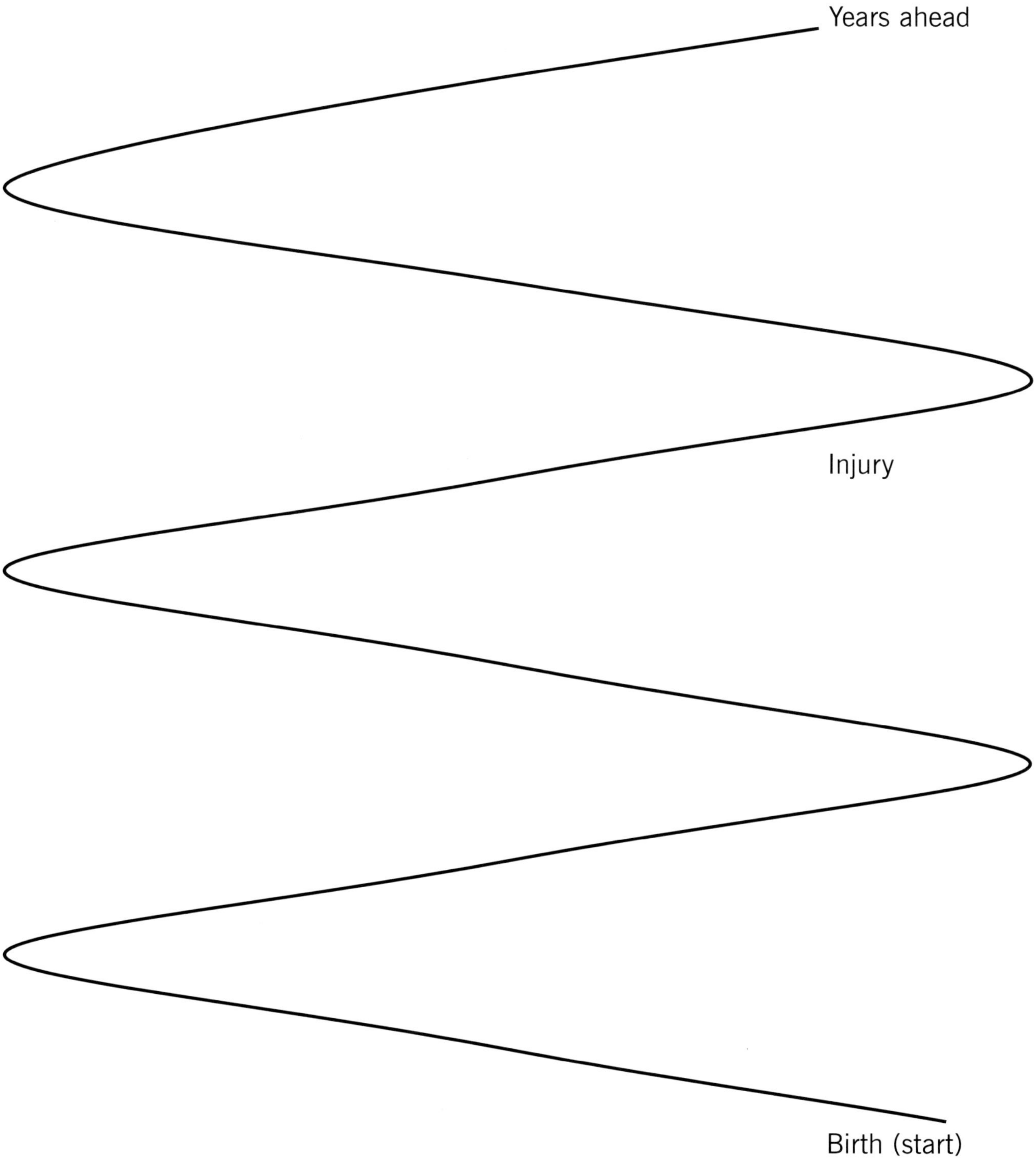

How did you find this exercise? Easy ☐ OK ☐ Quite difficult ☐ Very difficult ☐

EXERCISE 7

Structuring your week

How difficult do you think you will find this exercise? Easy ☐ OK ☐ Quite difficult ☐ Very difficult ☐

Instruction

A common problem after head injury is difficulties structuring your time – finding activities to do that are stimulating but not too stressful. Sometimes not enough activity can lead to depression and too much activity can lead to stress. Fill in your weekly timetable.

Monday	**Tuesday**	**Wednesday**	**Thursday**	**Friday**
Morning				
Afternoon				
Evening				

Saturday	**Sunday**
Morning	
Afternoon	
Evening	

1 How do you feel about your weekly timetable? What would you like to add or take away?

2 Think of any other activities that you might be interested in, for example, Hobbies, Voluntary work, Courses etc.

How did you find this exercise? Easy ☐ OK ☐ Quite difficult ☐ Very difficult ☐

EXERCISE 8

To tell or not to tell?

How difficult do you think you will find this exercise? Easy ☐ OK ☐ Quite difficult ☐ Very difficult ☐

Instruction

1 How easy do you find it to tell others about your brain injury and subsequent difficulties?

Easy ☐ OK ☐ Quite difficult ☐ Very difficult ☐

2

> **Chris's story**
> Chris is a 23-year-old single man who had a severe brain injury five years ago. He has made a good recovery, but still has some problems with memory, executive skills, fatigue, and lowered tolerance. For the last 18 months he has worked for a small computer company in a telesales job. He enjoys the job, but finds that to keep up he has to work long hours, sometimes takes work home, and is feeling increasingly stressed. He has a good relationship with his manager, but has not told him about his brain injury. His manager and colleagues have noticed that he is forgetful, has some difficulty prioritising and structuring his work, is less efficient and works late most evenings.

What are the advantages and disadvantages of telling his manager about his hidden disability?

Advantages
➤
➤
➤

Disadvantages
➤
➤
➤

3 Rate how likely it is that people would say the following things if you told them the full nature of your difficulties. 0 = not at all likely, 10 = very likely. Discuss.

Negative reactions	Rating
'Brain injury – you must be retarded – I see you completely differently now.'	
'You should be over it by now – you're swinging the lead.'	
'You're just looking for sympathy.'	
Add your own:	

Positive reactions	Rating
'I'm glad you've told me, now we can find ways of helping you more.'	
'I thought there was something wrong. I'm glad I know what it is now.'	
'That's OK, we're all struggling with something – I like your honesty.'	
Add your own:	

4 What is the best way of telling people about your difficulties? What words might you use?

How did you find this exercise? Easy ☐ OK ☐ Quite difficult ☐ Very difficult ☐

Disinhibition and lowered tolerance

How difficult do you think you will find this exercise? Easy ☐ OK ☐ Quite difficult ☐ Very difficult ☐

Instruction

Clare's story

I was at a dancing class with a friend last night. We were talking about the teacher, and my friend said she thought he was a good dancer. I said I did not think he was a good teacher. She did not seem to understand the point that I was making, and so I repeated myself, but considerably louder and in a rather angry voice. She was upset, because she could see that I was angry by the tone of my voice. Since my brain injury, I just don't seem to be able to mask my intolerance or keep it in – it just slips out. It's like somebody flicks a switch. I used to be much more in control of my emotions – now I feel like a child, but embarrassed. I really don't like the person that I've become, and I don't know how to deal with myself.

1 The above story illustrates the subtle problem of lowered tolerance and disinhibition after brain injury. Can you think of a situation where you have responded in a disinhibited way, or when your emotions have just 'slipped out' and caused trouble?

2 The lady in the story had a so-called 'minor brain injury' three years ago, and has no physical signs of disability. Can you suggest ways in which she could deal with the situation? Discuss the pros and cons of telling her friend that her outburst might be related to her accident.

How did you find this exercise? Easy ☐ OK ☐ Quite difficult ☐ Very difficult ☐

EXERCISE 10

Changing values

How difficult do you think you will find this exercise? Easy ☐ OK ☐ Quite difficult ☐ Very difficult ☐

Instruction

A brain injury is a life-changing event and affects the way we view ourselves, our view of the world, and our values.

1 Comment on the story below in terms of the individual's changed values.

John's story

I find that I am less controlling or planning of the future – more loose and personable. For example, I invited a group of different friends to the WOMAD music festival, some of whom knew each other and some who didn't. Before, I wouldn't have done that, or I'd have worried how they would get on with each other. Now I'm more easygoing and live more for the moment. I find myself saying, 'It was meant to be', or 'Whatever will be will be.'

2 Fill in the questionnaire below and discuss.

	Values	Agree	Disagree
a	I appreciate the moment more, and am less concerned with planning for the future.		
b	I value my friends and family more.		
c	I am more tolerant and accepting of others with a disability.		
d	I am less ambitious, materialistic and concerned with money.		
e	I recognise my own inner strength and sense of self more.		

3 Which of your attitudes or values has changed since your injury?

How did you find this exercise? Easy ☐ OK ☐ Quite difficult ☐ Very difficult ☐

EXERCISE 11

Changing roles

How difficult do you think you will find this exercise? Easy ☐ OK ☐ Quite difficult ☐ Very difficult ☐

Instruction

One of the most difficult things to adjust to after a brain injury is the change in roles that you and your family members have to make. Look at the following two examples, and then fill in the questionnaire about yourself.

'I used to be the irritable, prejudiced, black-and-white thinking and intolerant one in our relationship, and Marita used to be the angel who calmed me down. Since Marita's head injury we have swapped roles, and she is all those things. I don't know how I will cope.'

'I used to be the one that people would come to for advice, both at home and at work. My children would say, 'Dad, what do you think of this?' Now they don't any more.'

	Roles	Reduced or lost	Increased
1	Breadwinner, provider, or chief source of income		
2	Organiser of social activities such as holidays, outings, parties		
3	Bill-payer and organiser of finances		
4	Joker, quick-witted – life and soul of the party		
5	Advisor, source of advice and wise counsel		
6	'Calmer of troubled waters' – calms, soothes and settles a crisis		
7	Domestic – shopper, cooker, cleaner		
8	Handyman – adept at carrying out DIY and odd jobs		
9	Energiser – full of energy, ideas and 'get up and go'		

Identify the major roles that you feel you have lost, or that have been reduced since your injury.

➤

➤

Identify any new roles that you feel you have gained since your injury.

➤

➤

How do you feel about these role changes?

How did you find this exercise? Easy ☐ OK ☐ Quite difficult ☐ Very difficult ☐

Dependency

How difficult do you think you will find this exercise? Easy ☐ OK ☐ Quite difficult ☐ Very difficult ☐

Instruction

Immediately after a brain injury, you are likely to be very dependent on medical staff, nursing staff and family. Gradually you become more independent and start taking more responsibility. It is useful to assess in what areas of life you may be independent or dependent, and to identify areas where perhaps you could be more independent.

1 Complete the following rating scale.

Activity	**Completely independent**	**Slightly dependent**	**Dependent on others**
I travel on public transport.			
I go to the shops and do the shopping.			
I prepare and cook a meal for myself and others.			
I carry out household maintenance, such as decorating and routine car maintenance.			
I carry out social activities with friends, such as going to the cinema, pub, or restaurant.			
I manage the household bills, banking, and household accounts.			
I carry out household chores, such as vacuuming, cleaning and making the beds.			
I organise social events and holidays for myself and others.			

2 Select a task in which you think you could become more independent. Write down specific steps or goals that you can complete towards achieving this.

How did you find this exercise? Easy ☐ OK ☐ Quite difficult ☐ Very difficult ☐

Goal-planning 1

How difficult do you think you will find this exercise? Easy ☐ OK ☐ Quite difficult ☐ Very difficult ☐

Instruction

The following exercise is a useful way to loosen up your thinking, help you identify core values, and put you in a positive frame of mind for goal-planning. Answer each question as quickly as possible in the allotted time.

1 What five basic values in life are most important to you? (for example: friendship, money, etc)

Time allowed = 60 seconds

2 What are your three most important life goals?

Time allowed = 30 seconds

3 What would you do if you had six months to live?

Time allowed = 30 seconds

4 How would you change your life if you became an instant millionaire?

Time allowed = 30 seconds

5 What activities give you the greatest feeling of importance and satisfaction?

Time allowed = 60 seconds

6 What have you always wanted to do, but been afraid to attempt?

Time allowed = 30 seconds

How did you find this exercise? Easy ☐ OK ☐ Quite difficult ☐ Very difficult ☐

Goal-planning 2

How difficult do you think you will find this exercise? Easy ☐ OK ☐ Quite difficult ☐ Very difficult ☐

Instruction

1	*Write down two specific, well-defined goals to work towards over the next 12 months.* **Goal 1:** **Goal 2:**

2	Goal 1	*Identify five steps necessary to achieve that goal (the things you have to do).*	*Identify two potential obstacles.*
		➤ ➤ ➤ ➤ ➤	➤ ➤

3	Goal 2	*Identify five steps necessary to achieve that goal.*	*Identify two potential obstacles.*
		➤ ➤ ➤ ➤ ➤	➤ ➤

How did you find this exercise? Easy ☐ OK ☐ Quite difficult ☐ Very difficult ☐

Returning to work 1

How difficult do you think you will find this exercise? Easy ☐ OK ☐ Quite difficult ☐ Very difficult ☐

Instruction

1 Any job can be broken down into different component skills. Identify the three main components, or key skills, of your last job before your injury. Use the following list as a starter, but add your own if necessary.

Physical strength	Stamina	Dexterity	Travelling
Ability to learn	Multi-tasking,	Planning and organising	Problem-solving
Quick thinking	Time pressure	Decision-making	Coping with stress
Working in a team	Long hours	Motivating myself	Supervising others

➤ Key skill one:

➤ Key skill two:

➤ Key skill three:

2 Identify the three main problems caused by your injury, which are likely to cause you difficulties at work. The following list is a starter, but add your own if necessary.

Memory	Tiredness and fatigue	Multi-tasking	Planning and organising
Speech and talking	Speed of thinking	Short temper	Careless mistakes
Visual-perceptual	More emotional	Managing stress	Disinhibited/ impulsive

➤ Problem one:

➤ Problem two:

➤ Problem three:

3 Identify the three characteristics of your ideal job that you think might suit you. Again, the following list is to give you some ideas:

Something familiar	Few time pressures	Structure and routine
Little new learning	A sympathetic manager	One thing at a time
Good supervision	Interesting work	Short hours

➤ Characteristic one:

➤ Characteristic two:

➤ Characteristic three:

How did you find this exercise? Easy ☐ OK ☐ Quite difficult ☐ Very difficult ☐

Returning to work 2

How difficult do you think you will find this exercise? Easy ☐ OK ☐ Quite difficult ☐ Very difficult ☐

Instruction

1 Rank in order which of these problems would be the biggest obstacle to getting a part-time job (1 = biggest obstacle; 6 = least obstacle):

A slight weakness in the left leg, unable to walk long distances	
A tendency to tire more easily	
Poor insight and awareness of problems – 'there is nothing wrong with me'	
A mildly to moderately impaired memory	
A lowered tolerance and tendency to get angry more quickly	
A loss of sense of smell and taste	

2 Rank in order which of these jobs might be most suitable for a person who has had a brain injury and has moderate problems with memory, executive skills (doing lots of things at the same time and making decisions), speed of processing information, and lowered tolerance.

Managing Director of small company	
Sales-person for computer software company	
Working in the cataloguing section of the Meteorological Office library	
Working on the counter at a fast-food restaurant	
Working in a garden centre looking after the plants	

3 Identify three kinds of job that you could do, taking into account the residual difficulties that you have as a result of your brain injury.

How did you find this exercise? Easy ☐ OK ☐ Quite difficult ☐ Very difficult ☐

Work after a brain injury

How difficult do you think you will find this exercise? Easy ☐ OK ☐ Quite difficult ☐ Very difficult ☐

Instruction

Success at work has been conceptualised as having four basic ingredients:

- **Cooperativeness**: willing and able to work with others – to be able to postpone your own gratification to complete a job
- **Reliability**: to do what you say you will do – to follow through responsibilities
- **Effectiveness**: must be able to do the job
- **Efficiency**: to be able to complete the job at a rate that others would regard as normal

1 Using the model below, identify how your neuropsychological problems may interfere with the four ingredients of work productivity. Jot down relevant personal factors, or residual symptoms, by each side of the box.

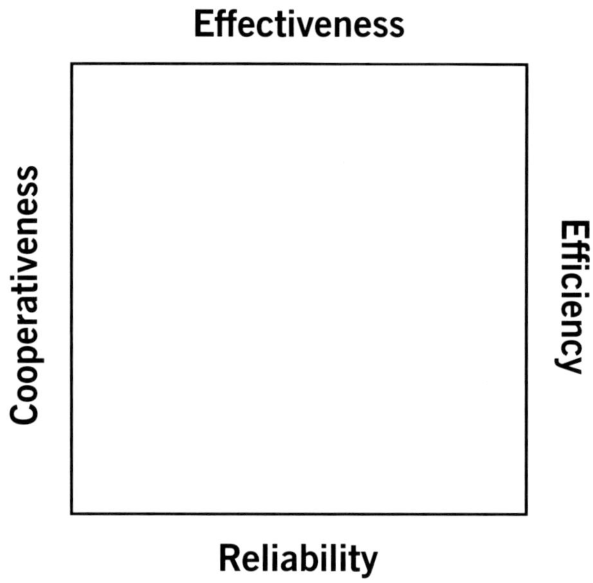

2 What are the main issues for you regarding a return to work, or your present working practice?

How did you find this exercise? Easy ☐ OK ☐ Quite difficult ☐ Very difficult ☐

'What's your advice?'

How difficult do you think you will find this exercise? Easy ☐ OK ☐ Quite difficult ☐ Very difficult ☐

Instruction
Imagine that you meet somebody who has recently had a brain injury, and they ask for your advice on how to cope with adjusting to life afterwards. This exercise helps you decide what you would and would not say.

1 Rank these statements in order, in terms of which is the best and worst advice (1 = best; 5 = worst). Discuss.

'Stay positive, there are always people worse off than yourself.'	
'The road to recovery takes time – don't be impatient.'	
'Get involved with a head injury support group like Headway.'	
'You can still do most things that you like, but you have to do them differently.'	
'You're lucky to be alive.'	

2 *What is the best advice you would give to somebody who has just had a brain injury? Write two statements that you would suggest might be good advice (these might or might not be similar to the ones above).*

➤

➤

3 *What is the worst thing that you can think off to say to somebody who has just had a brain injury, or what was the worst thing anybody said to you?*

How did you find this exercise? Easy ☐ OK ☐ Quite difficult ☐ Very difficult ☐

Maintaining quality relationships

How difficult do you think you will find this exercise? Easy ☐ OK ☐ Quite difficult ☐ Very difficult ☐

Instruction

After any brain injury, it is not just the individual who suffers, but usually the whole family - spouse, boy/girlfriends, and friends are affected. Relationships generally suffer. This exercise is aimed at examining the things you do that can either damage or help your relationships.

1 Identify a particular relationship with someone you are very close to – for example, friend, father, son, etc.

____

2 Rank in order which behaviour is most likely to improve your relationship. (1 = most positive; 6 = most negative.)

1 Openly expressing feelings of affection and love.	
2 Denying that you have any problems. This means you minimise difficulties, blame others, and refuse to talk about your real problems.	
3 Frequently expressing statements and feelings of 'gratitude' to the other for 'putting up with me'.	
4 Being as independent as possible – having an independent social life, hobbies, and possibly some form of work.	
5 Frequently losing your temper and becoming aggressive.	
6 Being relaxed and extremely laid back, and never worrying about anything.	

3 *Identify one kind of behaviour that you display now, that tends to irritate or upset other people, or those closest to you.*

4 *What one positive thing could you do that would improve the quality of your relationship?*

How did you find this exercise? Easy ☐ OK ☐ Quite difficult ☐ Very difficult ☐

Relationship changes

How difficult do you think you will find this exercise? Easy ☐ OK ☐ Quite difficult ☐ Very difficult ☐

Eric, aged 54, had a head injury five years ago and has an array of subtle hidden problems. He lives with his wife Jane who feels that their relationship has completely changed. She made the following statement:

"Eric is a completely different person from the man I married 30 years ago. People don't realize that I have lost the old Eric – he looks fine and superficially is okay for a while. But we are no longer equal partners, we don't jointly talk and make decisions together. I look after all the bills and finances now. I feel on my own because I've got nobody to plan things with or to share things. He no longer offers a shoulder for me to cry on; in fact he doesn't recognize or notice my moods. He is very preoccupied with himself. Recently the priest, whom I was very close to died and Eric didn't appear to feel anything and could not comfort me. If we watch a film together it is difficult to discuss it – he is very concrete in his thinking and misses anything subtle. He loses his temper quickly and gets jealous if I am away for too long. Worst of all he thinks 'there is nothing wrong with me".

1 Put yourself in Jane's shoes. From her brief statement identify three main losses for Jane within their relationship.

➤

➤

➤

2 Think about your main emotional relationship – with either your partner, a family member, or a friend. Put yourselves in their shoes and complete the following exercise.

I am ____________. I am ____________'s partner, parent, child, sibling, friend. (circle one) Since his/her injury our relationship is different in the following three ways.

➤

➤

➤

How did you find this exercise? Easy ☐ OK ☐ Quite difficult ☐ Very difficult ☐

Maintaining intimate relationships

How difficult do you think you will find this exercise? Easy ☐ OK ☐ Quite difficult ☐ Very difficult ☐

Instruction

After brain injury, there is a high rate of divorce and separation. Research suggests that non-injured spouses find a specific number of behaviours particularly difficult to cope with. To maintain relationships, these problems need to be identified, discussed and worked on. Mark on the table below if you recognise that you have any of the following tendencies.

Potential problems to relationships as suggested by research	**Do I have this tendency?** *No*	*Slight*	*Yes*	**Suggestions to work on**
1 I have become dependent – not carrying out activities on my own (work, social life, hobbies).				Stay as independent as possible – for example, attempt some form of work, or go to Headway – work at maintaining independent social life.
2 I do not express how I really feel. One wife said, 'I just don't know how he really feels.'				Try to talk openly about how you feel. If you have 'emotional flattening' and do not have strong feelings, talk about that.
3 I have a lowered tolerance – having angry explosive outbursts, irritability and socially inappropriate behavior.				Recognise that it is a real problem, and show that you are trying to do something about it. Discuss coping strategies. See a therapist. Do not deny the problem.
4 I make excessive statements of gratitude – for example, 'thank you for staying with me'.				Express appreciation for things that your partner does, but not in a self-pitying way.
5 I have a lack of insight and awareness – denying problems.				Talk to others. Face up and accept the changes. Listen to feedback.
6 I have apathy, and a lack of drive, or initiative. Never getting things done – being too laid back.				Recognise that this is a problem. Work out ways of coping, such as structuring your day, writing down goals, making action plans.

What other specific problems might jeopardise your relationship, and what one practical things can you do to alter this?

How did you find this exercise? Easy ☐ OK ☐ Quite difficult ☐ Very difficult ☐

Looking on the positive side

How difficult do you think you will find this exercise? Easy ☐ OK ☐ Quite difficult ☐ Very difficult ☐

Instruction

Any kind of brain injury is a life-changing event, with many negative consequences and losses. However, people do say that there are also some positive aspects to the experience: 'Every cloud has a silver lining.'

1 Below is a list of positive outcomes of brain injury that other people have suggested. Identify those with which you agree, and those with which you disagree.

Positive outcomes	Agree	Disagree
I am closer to certain members of my family.		
I am a more relaxed, laidback person.		
Because I no longer work, I have more time to myself.		
I am a nicer person.		
I am more conscious of living for today, rather than planning for tomorrow.		
I am a more sympathetic person regarding others with a disability.		

2 Identify three positive aspects to your injury, irrespective of how small. It does not matter if they are the same as in the above table.

3 Discuss as a group.

How did you find this exercise? Easy ☐ OK ☐ Quite difficult ☐ Very difficult ☐

Common misconceptions

How difficult do you think you will find this exercise? Easy ☐ OK ☐ Quite difficult ☐ Very difficult ☐

Instruction

1 The following questionnaire was given to members of the public. The results suggest that the general public have many misconceptions about brain injury. Fill in the questionnaire, and see how you get on.

		True (T) or False (F)
1	Wearing seat belts causes as many injuries as it prevents.	
2	A brain injury can cause brain damage, even if the person is not knocked out.	
3	A little brain damage doesn't matter much, as people only use part of their brains anyway.	
4	Most people with brain injury are not fully aware of the effects on their behaviour.	
5	When people are knocked unconscious, most people wake up quickly with no lasting effects.	
6	Breast cancer is more common than brain injury.	
7	A person with a brain injury will have more difficulty remembering things from the past than in learning new things.	
8	Sometimes a second blow to the head can help a person remember things that were forgotten.	
9	People who have had one brain injury are more likely to have a second one.	
10	Once the person with the brain injury feels 'back to normal', the recovery process is complete.	
11	Complete recovery from a very severe brain injury is not possible, no matter how much the person wants to recover.	
12	Drinking alcohol usually affects a person differently after a brain injury.	

2 Make up one statement about a specific aspect of brain injury, from your own experience, that the general public might struggle to be aware of.

How did you find this exercise? Easy ☐ OK ☐ Quite difficult ☐ Very difficult ☐

Dealing with misconceptions

How difficult do you think you will find this exercise? Easy ☐ OK ☐ Quite difficult ☐ Very difficult ☐

Instruction

Most people know little of the reality of brain injury. In one survey, 50 per cent of the sample thought that you just wake up and are left with no residual problems. People often say things like: 'You look well – there is nothing wrong with you'.

1 Write down a list of comments that people have made to you that are typical misconceptions, showing how little they understand about brain injury.

What do you say to other people to explain some of your difficulties? Many people avoid certain words or phrases, such as 'brain damage', preferring a less stigmatised term, such as 'head injury.' One man said, 'I had a knock and am now much slower.'

2 Write down a statement you might use to explain your difficulties.

3 Identify words or phrases that you do not like or would not use. Discuss.

How did you find this exercise? Easy ☐ OK ☐ Quite difficult ☐ Very difficult ☐

Coping with depression

How difficult do you think you will find this exercise? Easy ☐ OK ☐ Quite difficult ☐ Very difficult ☐

Instruction

Most of us get depressed or low at times. This exercise looks at two important skills in coping. One is to recognise the things, or triggers, that are likely to lead to depression – for example, being inactive, being isolated, having arguments, etc. The second is to deliberately employ a method of coping – or to deliberately do something that makes us feel better – for example, arrange an activity; talk to someone; write down thoughts.

1 Identify things that make you feel depressed.

2 Identify things you can do to make yourself feel less depressed.

How did you find this exercise? Easy ☐ OK ☐ Quite difficult ☐ Very difficult ☐

EXERCISE 26

Thinking and depression

How difficult do you think you will find this exercise? Easy ☐ OK ☐ Quite difficult ☐ Very difficult ☐

Instruction

Certain ways of thinking, or particular thoughts, can make us feel either good about ourselves or bad about ourselves. If you are prone to depression, it is useful to identify and challenge those negative thoughts that are 'bringing you down'.

1 Complete the following rating scale, marking how often you experience the following thoughts:

Negative Thoughts	**Frequently**	**Sometimes**	**Rarely**
My life has been ruined.			
Before my injury life was so much better.			
I can't do anything, achieve anything, or enjoy anything.			
I will never be able to work, or do anything productive again.			
I am a burden to my family and friends.			

2

Identify your top negative thought – for example, 'I can't do anything with my life.'	Identify positive challenges to these thoughts – for example, 'I can do lots of things, but the challenge is that I have to do them differently.'

3 Identify two positive thoughts that lift your mood – for example, 'Compared to how I was immediately after my injury, I'm doing very well.'

How did you find this exercise? Easy ☐ OK ☐ Quite difficult ☐ Very difficult ☐

EXERCISE 27

Challenging negative thoughts

How difficult do you think you will find this exercise? Easy ☐ OK ☐ Quite difficult ☐ Very difficult ☐

Instruction

We are all prone to negative thoughts at times. These often enter our minds as very 'black and white', catastrophic statements, that on close examination are simply not true. Make up positive challenges to the negative thoughts below.

	Thought	Positive Challenge
1	Why did it happen to me?	
2	I can't do anything.	
3	I am a burden to everybody – no use to anybody.	
4	I've got to get back to exactly how I was.	
5	My life is ruined.	
6	Add your own negative thoughts.	

How did you find this exercise? Easy ☐ OK ☐ Quite difficult ☐ Very difficult ☐

Things that 'wind me up'

How difficult do you think you will find this exercise? Easy ☐ OK ☐ Quite difficult ☐ Very difficult ☐

Instruction

In order to learn some ways of controlling temper it is important to identify the subtle triggers that 'wind' us up. These are often things that people do or say. Look at the two examples below and then try to think of some situations that 'wind you up'. Then fill in the right hand column that focuses on the reasons why this is so annoying.

	Situations that 'wind me up' – what others do or say	**What is it about this that is so annoying**
1	My wife reminds me to take my medication, or reminds me to brush my teeth.	I feel like a child in the way she speaks to me. It reminds me of my problems, which I'd rather forget. My pride is dented.
2	More than one person talking at the same time in a group.	I can't follow what people say. I can't switch my attention as well. I feel inadequate and left out.
3		
4		

Identify any ways that you could cope with any of the above situations better.

How did you find this exercise? Easy ☐ OK ☐ Quite difficult ☐ Very difficult ☐

Anger: identifying the triggers

How difficult do you think you will find this exercise? Easy ☐ OK ☐ Quite difficult ☐ Very difficult ☐

Instruction

After brain injury, you often have a lowered tolerance of frustration. This is due to injury of the frontal areas of the brain. Anger management has two main components: (1) Identifying the triggers – the situations that wind you up; (2) Learning to cope with those situations and your thoughts and feelings.

1 Identify five of the following situations that you recognise as triggers to your anger. Rate them in order of 1–5 (1 = happens most often).

	Ranking
Noise: High levels of background noise	
Tiredness: Feeling tired and fatigued	
Alcohol: Having drunk alcohol	
Forgetting 'silly little things' and making careless mistakes	
Feeling left out – unable to keep up in conversations – being ignored	
Feeling that I am being told off – treated like a child – patronised	
Conflict: People disagreeing with me – not falling in line with what I want	
Feeling bored – having nothing to do that is stimulating	
Stress and time-pressure overload: build-up of stresses – too much to do and too little time – feeling unable to cope	
Being kept waiting – impatient – 'I want it now'	
Any other – describe:	

2 Identify a recent situation where you lost your temper. What were the triggers? What were the thoughts that went through your head at the time? Discuss.

Situation/Trigger:

Thoughts:

How did you find this exercise? Easy ☐ OK ☐ Quite difficult ☐ Very difficult ☐

Anger: ways of coping

How difficult do you think you will find this exercise? Easy ☐ OK ☐ Quite difficult ☐ Very difficult ☐

Instruction

The left-hand column contains a list of situations or common 'triggers to anger'. The right-hand column lists a number of 'coping strategies'. Match the appropriate coping strategy to the appropriate trigger. Put the letter of the coping strategy in the middle column.

	Triggers to anger	*Write in letter that fits trigger*		**Coping strategy**
1	Drinking too much alcohol		A	Forgive yourself – next time write it down.
2	Feeling tired		B	Plan activities that are interesting for the future.
3	A noisy, chaotic environment		C	Say, 'We'll have to agree to differ.'
4	Forgetting something trivial		D	Say, 'I feel like a child when you speak to me like that.'
5	Feeling left out of a conversation with your family		E	Say 'No' – be assertive. Tell people that you simply cannot manage too many things.
6	Feeling bored – nothing to do		F	Think of yourself as being flexible – shrug your shoulders – take a deep breath.
7	Being kept waiting		G	Pace yourself – take a sleep in the day if necessary.
8	Somebody disagreeing with your opinion		H	Say, 'I am feeling left out' – make a joke of it.
9	Being spoken to in a patronising way – like a child		I	Drink non-alcoholic drinks.
10	Somebody does something that means a last-minute change of your plans		J	Say to yourself 'There is nothing I can do' – treat as an opportunity to practise relaxation.
11	Being overloaded with demands and requests from others		K	Explain that you 'cannot filter out background noise'. Turn something off.

Identify one other trigger to your anger and your way of coping.

How did you find this exercise? Easy ☐ OK ☐ Quite difficult ☐ Very difficult ☐

Ways of managing your temper

How difficult do you think you will find this exercise? Easy ☐ OK ☐ Quite difficult ☐ Very difficult ☐

Instruction

Most types of brain injury leave the injured person with a lowered tolerance of frustration, and a tendency to get angry more quickly. This can often be a major disability. Look at this list of coping strategies, and identify which ones you use.

		Tick if used
1	**Identify the triggers**. Recognise the situations that wind you up, then either avoid them, or work out a better way of coping, but be prepared.	
2	**Breathing exercises**. Calm yourself by taking deep breaths from your stomach, not your chest. Focus on breathing out slowly.	
3	**Count to ten**. Simple, but a good distraction. Count and speak slowly.	
4	**Positive self-statements**. Identify key words that you can say to yourself under your breath in difficult situations – for example, 'Challenge – this is my biggest challenge'.	
5	**Visualise coping in difficult situations**. Prepare and rehearse how you will cope in difficult situations. Shut your eyes, and go through difficult scenarios.	
6	**Leave the situation.** If you feel you are 'losing it', remove yourself from the situation and calm down before returning.	
7	**Challenge your 'shoulds' and 'oughts'**. Examine the core beliefs behind your anger. It's not other people who make you angry; rather, it's the beliefs that you have in your head about how people should behave.	
8	**Manage your stress**. Plan your days so that you are not overwhelmed or too tired to cope – leave 'breathing spaces' – avoid an overload.	
9	**Learn a relaxation exercise**. Drop your shoulders, loosen your hands, use a relaxation tape or take up yoga.	
10	**Physical exercise.** Use up excess energy and adrenaline – stay fit.	
11	**Express the feeling beneath the anger**. Underneath anger is often a feeling of hurt, rejection, inadequacy or frustration. Tell the person you feel hurt.	
12	**Express yourself assertively**. Talk it out at the time, rather than bottling it up and allowing resentment to build. Practise saying, 'I am feeling angry because…'.	
13	**Distract yourself**. Busy yourself with something else, or think of something different.	
14	Add any other ways that might help with managing anger:	

How did you find this exercise? Easy ☐ OK ☐ Quite difficult ☐ Very difficult ☐

Facing fears and phobias

How difficult do you think you will find this exercise? Easy ☐ OK ☐ Quite difficult ☐ Very difficult ☐

Instruction

We all have fears and anxieties, or situations we avoid. After a head injury these may include; avoiding public transport, crossing the road, travelling, speaking on the phone, or going into social situations. The aim of this exercise is to identify a particular fear, then break it down, and work out a number of steps to overcome it.

Identify a situation that makes you feel anxious and that you avoid. Describe the situation in as much specific detail as possible, for example 'Travel alone on a number 17 bus into town on a Saturday morning'. Now rate how anxious that situation makes you on a scale of 0 – 10. (0 = no anxiety, 10 = extreme anxiety)

Identify a number of other situations, associated with your main feared situation, and rate how anxious they make you feel. (For example, walk to bus stop = 4, Go on bus with partner = 7, Catch bus for two stops on own = 8). Now create a hierarchy of situations rated in order of anxiety, with the easiest at the bottom and the hardest at the top. The task is to start on the easier ones and work up to the top until you have overcome your fear.

	Target Situations	Anxiety Rating 0–10
1	(most difficult)	
2		
3		
4		
5		
6		
7	(least difficult)	

How did you find this exercise? Easy ☐ OK ☐ Quite difficult ☐ Very difficult ☐

Dealing with fatigue

How difficult do you think you will find this exercise? Easy ☐ OK ☐ Quite difficult ☐ Very difficult ☐

Instruction

Becoming easily fatigued and tired are major problems after brain injury, particularly in the early stages. This is not due just to physical exertion, but also to mental effort and concentration. Your injured brain is saying 'I want to rest – I want a break', and it is important to heed that message rather than pushing yourself and hoping that it will just go away.

1 What happens to you if you 'overdo it', 'take on too much', or 'push yourself too far'? Break down your reaction into physical, mental and emotional changes.

Physical changes
Mental changes
Emotional and behavioural changes

2 Which of the following positive ways of managing fatigue do you use regularly?

	Yes	**Sometimes**	**No**
I am aware of the early warning signs that I am 'overdoing it'.			
I make a point of saying 'no' to requests that might be too demanding.			
I tend to pace myself – planning and structuring my time more.			
I take regular breaks to recharge my batteries.			
I sleep more, and if necessary will have a nap during the day.			

3 Identify any other ways that you manage your fatigue.

How did you find this exercise? Easy ☐ OK ☐ Quite difficult ☐ Very difficult ☐

Changing focus

How difficult do you think you will find this exercise? Easy ☐ OK ☐ Quite difficult ☐ Very difficult ☐

Instruction

It has been said that meaning and satisfaction in life come from three sources – work, loving relationships and play. These are often areas that are disrupted after a brain injury. It is important to accept that such life changes occur, and that things have to be done differently. For example: Peter enjoyed photography, but could not use his damaged right hand to press the button on his camera, so he now holds his camera upside down and uses his left hand. Lisa enjoyed painting, but after her accident she had a tremor, which she managed to build into her work, giving it a vibrant sensation. Adaptation can be positive – a new source of creative achievement.

1 **Play:** *Identify an important enjoyable activity or hobby, and look at how you could still do it, but differently or with a change of focus.*

2 **Work:** *Identify an area of work that interests you, in which you could involve yourself with a change of focus.*

How did you find this exercise? Easy ☐ OK ☐ Quite difficult ☐ Very difficult ☐

EXERCISE 35

Friendship after brain injury

How difficult do you think you will find this exercise? Easy ☐ OK ☐ Quite difficult ☐ Very difficult ☐

Instruction

Answer the questions, and then discuss as a group.

1 Research suggests that after a significant brain injury, people tend to lose contact with old friends. Write down some of the reasons why this might be so.

➤

➤

2 How do you be a friend to somebody who has had a brain injury? List some 'dos' and 'don'ts'.

Dos	Don'ts

3 What are your strengths and weakness as a friend?

Strengths	Weaknesses

4 Try making an A–Z of friendship: A friend is someone who ...
Accepts your failings. **B**elieves in you. **C**alls for any reason.
Doesn't let people run you down...

E...	F...	G...
H...	I...	J...
K...	L...	M...
N...	O...	P...
Q...	R...	S...
T...	U...	V...
W...	Y...	Z...

How did you find this exercise? Easy ☐ OK ☐ Quite difficult ☐ Very difficult ☐

Asking for help – an 'enabler'

How difficult do you think you will find this exercise? Easy ☐ OK ☐ Quite difficult ☐ Very difficult ☐

Instruction

1 For some people, asking for help can be a difficult thing to do. There seems to be a fine balance between asking for too much help, and unassertively not asking for any help. How do you view yourself? Answer the following questions and discuss:

	Agree	**Disagree**
I hate being dependant on others or asking for help.		
I accept that I need help in certain situations.		
I can openly ask for help without feeling bad about it.		
I get so much help that I am losing my ability and my desire to do things for myself.		

2 Some people have an 'enabler', or a type of carer who helps you to do things that you would not normally be able to do. One man had two part-time enablers; one was interested in music and took him to concerts, and the other was interested in sport and fitness and took him on outdoor activities. Imagine if you were offered an enabler. Draw up a list of activities that you would like to attempt – or have help with – with the aid of the enabler. These are activities that you need some help with.

➤

➤

➤

➤

➤

How did you find this exercise? Easy ☐ OK ☐ Quite difficult ☐ Very difficult ☐

Forgiving yourself

How difficult do you think you will find this exercise? Easy ☐ OK ☐ Quite difficult ☐ Very difficult ☐

Instruction

Ellie, aged twenty-six, had a serious head injury five years ago but was managing to hold down a job as an administrative assistant at an army base. She was highly motivated to do a good job and hated to make mistakes. However, because of her head injury she was more forgetful and did make the occasional careless error. Every time this happened she would either get angry with herself, or angry with others, and then become miserable and depressed. She recognised that she needed to be easier on herself and be more forgiving of herself.

Below are a list of self-statements Ellie could make to herself to feel less angry and depressed and to forgive herself. Number in order your top three statements which you think might be most useful to Ellie – these will probably be statements that you would make to yourself.

1	We all make mistakes, nobody is perfect	
2	I didn't mean to and I am trying my hardest	
3	I have made good progress since my accident and I am still improving	
4	I am disappointed but it is only one aspect of me – one part of my life	
5	I need to lower my expectations – life is more difficult with a brain injury	
6	I'll feel better tomorrow – time is a great healer	
7	It is not the end of the world, there are more important things in life	
	Add your own forgiving thoughts	

1 Describe a situation where because of your injury, you made a mistake, forgot something, did something embarrassing or lost your temper more quickly and then felt bad about it afterwards.

2 Identify two key 'forgiving thoughts' that might be appropriate to your situation – thoughts that make you feel better.

➤

➤

How did you find this exercise? Easy ☐ OK ☐ Quite difficult ☐ Very difficult ☐

The hero's journey

How difficult do you think you will find this exercise? Easy ☐ OK ☐ Quite difficult ☐ Very difficult ☐

Instruction

The notion of the 'hero's journey' is embedded in most cultures and world religions, whether it is Jesus Christ, Ulysses, or Buddha, and it is a very apt metaphor for understanding life after brain injury. The journey involves a number of stages: first, leaving the security of home with all its certainties; second, facing the things that scare you most; third, using cunning and bravery to overcome your fears; fourth, returning home by a different way. Think about how this applies to your life.

1 What are you leaving behind – your major losses that you are letting go of (for example, career, relationships, hobbies)?

2 Facing what scares you most. What are the things that you have to face that scare you most (for example, failing; not being able to work; the reaction of others)?

3 What specific things do you do to cope with these challenges (for example, look back on my progress since the accident; use humour; carry a diary)?

4 Returning home to comfort and security by another way. What is the different way? What is your new way forwards towards security? Where are you hoping to settle?

How did you find this exercise? Easy ☐ OK ☐ Quite difficult ☐ Very difficult ☐

Quality of life

How difficult do you think you will find this exercise? Easy ☐ OK ☐ Quite difficult ☐ Very difficult ☐

Instruction

Answer the questions, and then discuss as a group.

1 Quality of life means different things to each of us. It is sometimes used to describe an overall sense of well-being, or how good life is. When asked, 'What makes life worth living, or what gives a life quality?', these are some of the things people say. Try to put these in order for yourself, by marking a number next to each one (1 = very important; 2 = important; 3 = not important).

Family		Holidays		Sex life	
Religion		A comfortable home		Friends	
A good job		Being physically healthy		Environment	
Money		Art and being creative		Social life	
Sport		Intimate relationships		Education	

2 When people have suffered a trauma like a brain injury, their priorities often change. Things previously taken for granted are valued much more. List two things that are more important to you now than they were before.

➤

➤

3 Work, love and play have been identified as three areas to guide people in recovery. Think about your week, and list your activities under these headings:

Work – something purposeful to do everyday

Love – friends, colleagues and relationships

Play – leisure, enjoying yourself, having fun

How did you find this exercise? Easy ☐ OK ☐ Quite difficult ☐ Very difficult ☐

Saying 'no' and delegating

How difficult do you think you will find this exercise? Easy ☐ OK ☐ Quite difficult ☐ Very difficult ☐

Instruction

After a brain injury, where you are aware that your abilities are now more limited, you need to be able to protect yourself from the demands of others who are less aware of your limitations. This is a vital skill, as if you cannot turn off the stress tap you will be easily overwhelmed.

Think of one situation where you have deliberately said no to a recent demand or delegated a task to somebody else.

Think of one situation which you would like to delegate or say no to.

People find it difficult to delegate and say no for a variety of reasons. Which do you identify with? Discuss.

		Tick if you agree
1	Saying no is rejecting somebody and they might feel hurt.	
2	Saying no is rude – you should always try to help others.	
3	Saying no is selfish.	
4	Delegating a task shows weakness – that I can't cope.	
5	I like to do things myself, it makes me feel in control and useful.	
6	I do not like imposing on others.	
7	Add your own:	

What are some of the advantages of delegating and saying no – for yourself and others?

How did you find this exercise? Easy ☐ OK ☐ Quite difficult ☐ Very difficult ☐

The stages of the grief process

How difficult do you think you will find this exercise? Easy ☐ OK ☐ Quite difficult ☐ Very difficult ☐

Instruction

Coming to terms with a brain injury is similar in some ways to coming to terms with a bereavement. People might go through stages of emotional reactions.

1 Look at the chart below, and mark off grieving stages that you have been through, and the stage where you are at now. There is no right or wrong: some people do not go through these stages or they may go in a different order.

The grief process		**Tick the stage you are at**
1 Denial	'I don't believe it. It hasn't happened', 'I'm going to be fine.' This stage may act as a buffer. The individual cannot handle the news, and therefore their only option is to deny it. Saying: 'I will be back to normal soon.' Family denies as well.	
2 Anger	Anger, resentment and rage are normal reactions to loss. Anger towards those responsible. Anger and frustration with self. 'Why me?'; 'If only…'	
3 Bargaining	Attempting to delay, or to reduce the effects of the loss. 'If I work hard my speech will come back.'	
4 Depression	Impairments can no longer be denied, and anger has been vented. Attempts to overcome losses have failed, leaving a greater sense of loss. The full impact of the reality of the situation results in natural depression.	
5 Acceptance	There is an acknowledgement of the reality. Recognising problems and new limitations, and talking about them openly. Learning to live with only a partial recovery and disabilities. 'My life is now very different.' Finding ways around the problems. Feeling more settled and being more able to plan.	

2 Identify what stages you have been through if your experience is different from the above?

How did you find this exercise? Easy ☐ OK ☐ Quite difficult ☐ Very difficult ☐

Tips for coping with adjustment

How difficult do you think you will find this exercise? Easy ☐ OK ☐ Quite difficult ☐ Very difficult ☐

Instruction

1 Emotional adjustment to life after brain injury means something like 'having understood and accepted what has happened, adjusted my lifestyle accordingly and no longer feel excessively emotionally distressed by my situation.' Rate how you think you are in terms of 'emotional adjustment'.

1	2	3	4	5
Poor adjustment		Reasonable adjustment		Good adjustment

2 Examine the list of tips or advice on coping with adjustment after brain injury, and identify which ones you would consider your top five tips. Rank them in order (1 = top; 5 = bottom). Are there any you would disagree with?

1	Understand what is going on. Look for information in books, ask questions. Improve your awareness.	
2	Meet other people in a similar situation. Don't isolate yourself.	
3	Be patient – the road towards recovery and adjustment is a long, long road.	
4	Set goals for yourself – little steps to make gains – 'where there is a will there is a way'. Don't give up.	
5	Be kind to yourself – pace yourself. Forgive yourself when you make a mistake.	
6	Monitor your progress since your injury – appreciate how far you have come. Count your blessings.	
7	Accept your limitations and lower your expectations. You can still do anything you like, but you might have to do it differently.	
8	Learn to appreciate the moment, rather than racing ahead. Make the most of each day – you have been given a second chance.	
9	Learn to use strategies to cope with and compensate for your difficulties.	
10	Be assertive, learn to say no, delegate and tell people you have problems if appropriate.	

Add any other advice that you think might be helpful.

How did you find this exercise? Easy ☐ OK ☐ Quite difficult ☐ Very difficult ☐

What you say to yourself to make sense of it

How difficult do you think you will find this exercise? Easy ☐ OK ☐ Quite difficult ☐ Very difficult ☐

Instruction

Research suggests that people who make a good emotional adjustment to life after head injury or are 'at ease with themselves', tend to think in a particular way. The research looked at self-statements or self-narratives that people make – meaning what people say to themselves to make sense of their situation.

Which of the following self-statements fits in best with your experience? Rank the self-statements that you identify with in order from most to least. (Identify with most = 1, identify with least = 5). Discuss.

1	'Things could be worse – there are people worse off than me. I could have died – I count my blessings.'	
2	'I have grown as a person because of this. I am a stronger person, more resilient, more aware of my inner strength. I have been through something bad and conquered it.'	
3	'I am still making progress, working towards getting better, moving in a positive direction. I focus on the progress I have already made.'	
4	'I focus on the "here and now" and appreciate the moment much more, rather than constantly striving. One day at a time. I value people more.	
5	'I want to use my experiences to make things better – to channel my energy and do something constructive to help others.'	

Write your own self-statement or self-narrative in a sentence or two. This is something that you might say to youself to make sense of your experience of life after brain injury.

How did you find this exercise? Easy ☐ OK ☐ Quite difficult ☐ Very difficult ☐

Thinking Skills Exercise 4: Word association

Page 72

- ➤ Roll, sticky, clear = SELLOTAPE®
- ➤ Wrinkles, steam, clothes = WASHING MACHINE
- ➤ Feathers, black, fly = CROW
- ➤ Border, wood, post = FENCE
- ➤ Stripe, hooves, crossing = ZEBRA
- ➤ Metal, paper, cuts = SCISSORS
- ➤ Exhaust, ticket, travel = BUSES
- ➤ Wallet, plastic, signature = CREDIT-CARD
- ➤ Clothes, wet, peg = WASHING LINE
- ➤ Green, iron, card = GOLF
- ➤ Light, bulb, pavement = LAMP-POST
- ➤ Warm, water, pipe = DISHWASHER
- ➤ Hard, black, playtime = TARMAC
- ➤ Sugar, tin, rise = BAKING
- ➤ Blade, wood, adjust = PLANE
- ➤ Round, hole, cotton = BUTTON
- ➤ Soft, nose, pocket = BABY KANGAROO
- ➤ Water, visibility, mountain-top = MIST
- ➤ Pump, body, love = HEART
- ➤ Hot, space, god = SUN

Thinking Skills Exercise 6: Words with multiple meanings

Page 74

Word	First meaning	Second meaning	Third meaning
Spring	A season	To jump	A coil of metal
Blue	A colour	Sadness	Blowing air
Through	Passing beyond	Throwing something	
Plant	Heavy machinery	To put into the ground	A growing seedling
Right	A direction	An entitlement	A ritual
Table	To eat dinner off	To propose an idea	
Nail	A metal shard to hold things together	Part of the fingers and toes	To make sure you get someone
Bean	A foodstuff	Describing having visited somewhere	
Marble	A round glass ball	A kind of rock	A kind of art form
Step	A stair	To take a pace	A grade or level to attain or follow
Grass	The lawn	To reveal secrets	Cannabis
Bat	Played with in cricket	A flying mammal	To hit something
Train	To work hard at achieving – in sport	A means of transport	To force a plant or creeper to grow in a certain direction
Score	The amount of points	To gain a goal	To mark a fold in paper
Prize	To value something greatly	The reward given to the winner	To lever something off something else
Court	The playing area for tennis	To win someone's love	To catch something
Stick	A small piece of wood	To glue	

Thinking Skills Exercise 7: Analogies

Page 75

- ➤ Shoe is to foot as Glove is to HAND
- ➤ Lion is to jungle as Bat is to CAVE
- ➤ Mechanic is to car as Plumber is to PIPES
- ➤ Banana is to peel as Bread is to CUT
- ➤ Referee is to soccer as Umpire is to CRICKET/TENNIS
- ➤ Nail polish is to nail as Mascara is to EYES
- ➤ Gun is to bullet as Hose is to WATER
- ➤ Hair is to wig as Teeth are to MOUTH
- ➤ Ant is to nest as Bees are to HIVE
- ➤ Heart is to chest as Brain is to HEAD

- Guitar is to string as Piano is to KEYS
- Watch is to strap as Trousers are to BELT
- January is to winter as September is to AUTUMN/FALL
- The Koran is to Muslims as the Bible is to CHRISTIANS
- Cake is to baking as Carrots are to COOKING
- Driver is to car as Pilot is to PLANE
- General is to Army as Admiral is to NAVY

Thinking Skills Exercise 8: Odd one out — Page 76

By row: 2 Jane Pine Kangaroo New York Oboe Bat Rat Jewel Cola Saucer Cheque Tie Chicken Bicycle

Thinking Skills Exercise 9: Complete the word — Page 77

ENT	ENTRANCE	Way in
PUR	PURPLE	Colour
GIN	BEGIN	Start
MAN	MANCHESTER/MANHATTAN	City
PAT	PATTERN	Design
BAL	BALLOT	Vote
OPP	OPPOSITE	Completely different
NER	NERVOUS	Worried
SET	SETTLED	Calm
BAD	BADMINTON	Sport
USH	BRUSH	Used for painting
SON	PERSON	An individual
LET	TOILET	Ladies' room
EST	INVESTIGATE	Search
NER	CORNER	Bend
ENC	PENCIL	Something to write with
PHA	ELEPHANT	Big animal
BET	ALPHABET	Group of letters

Thinking Skills Exercise 10: Connections — Page 78

Cat	Hair	Allergy	A tissue
Grass	Cut	Knife	A murder
A tin of tuna	Fish	Cake	A party dress
One sock	Pair	Tree	House
A tie	Neck	Head	Soccer
A dead mouse	Trap	Door	Shed
Car	Crash	Tree	Oasis
A knife	Fork	Hay	Farm
Tony Blair	Leader	Judge	Wig
A postman	Letter	Bomb	Suicide

Thinking Skills Exercise 15: Correct interpretation — Page 83

The correct interpretations are:

1 If you start early you will be rewarded. = The early bird catches the worm.
3 If you are determined, you will succeed. = Where there's a will there's a way.
6 If too many people are involved, they get in each other's way. = Too many cooks spoil the broth.
8 If you do something for me, I will look after you. = One good turn deserves another.
9 Take advantage of an opportunity when it presents itself. = Strike while the iron is hot.
11 When one bad thing happens, another one follows close behind. = When it rains, it pours.
12 If somebody does not have a job it means they are lazy. = Don't judge a book by its cover.
16 He gets to the point of the discussion or issue quickly. = He hits the nail on the head.

Thinking Skills Exercise 17: Match the logos — Page 85

Number 1 is from logo 12 – Yellow Pages
Number 2 is from logo 4 – Ford
Number 3 is from logo 6 – Lego
Number 4 is from logo 3 – Penguin Books
Number 5 is from logo 1 – The National Lottery
Number 6 is from logo 8 – Adidas
Number 7 is from logo 11 – Pepsi
Number 8 is from logo 10 – Mercedes-Benz
Number 9 is from logo 5 – Paramount
Number 10 is from logo 2 – Levi's
Number 11 is from logo 7 – Ikea
Number 12 is from logo 9 – Channel 4

Thinking Skills Exercise 18: Match the traffic signs — Page 86

Section 1 is taken from traffic sign number 4
Section 2 is taken from traffic sign number 5
Section 3 is taken from traffic sign number 7
Section 4 is taken from traffic sign number 6
Section 5 is taken from traffic sign number 9
Section 6 is taken from traffic sign number 8
Section 7 is taken from traffic sign number 1
Section 8 is taken from traffic sign number 2
Section 9 is taken from traffic sign number 3

Thinking Skills Exercise 20: Embedded words 1 — Page 88

~~egg~~	rose	London	sellotape®	rock	~~fish~~	(zebra)	music	tissue	John	cat	glue
bright	super	fly	(American flag)	diamond	star	annual	switch	parrot	witch		
dance	Velcro	square	kitchen	(lined paper)	computer	holiday	~~ice cream~~	granite			
(barcode)	pen	grass	blue	four	granite	~~rabbit~~	pillow	~~ruler~~	swan	~~chicken~~	
~~Roman road~~	swerve	tennis	crow	bee	radiator	glass	cold	~~toffee~~	~~mutton~~		
mountain	(barber's pole)	silk	Africa	seaside	hair	paperclip	~~treacle~~	~~port~~	~~cola~~		
month	triangle	five	blanket	bed	silk	London	cloud	paper	water	pie	maths
subway	pomp	music	fur	(piano keyboard)	pills	~~beef~~	wallet	wrist	(tiger)	clown	
~~jam~~	~~milk~~	watch	sand	lake	bridge	kite	kitten	map	balloon	baboon	stick
~~carrot~~	hitch	club	~~light rays~~	broach	(wasp)	diamond	bath	~~melted cheese~~	(French flag)		
book	~~goat~~	wallpaper paste	square	bag	~~carrot~~	flipper	~~horizon~~	swimming	sock		
~~deer~~	brick	~~laser beam~~	hot tarmac	worm	ant	balloon	swear	kangaroo	nice		
radio	crash	underwear	~~honey~~	alphabet	car	(sergeant's chevrons)	~~curry~~				

The following words are mentioned twice: London, music, diamond, square, granite, silk, balloon, carrot

Thinking Skills Exercise 21: Embedded words 2 — Page 89

fire violin ~~Rome~~ sellotape® rock ~~bear~~ ~~zebra~~ sun tissue one ~~cat~~ glue
brimstone super mouse American flag diamond ~~York~~ switch ~~mole~~ witch dance
Velcro three kitchen burn computer holiday ice-cream note barcode pen grass
blue four granite ~~rabbit~~ pillow ruler ~~hen~~ scald Roman road swerve tennis
~~wolf~~ flame glass ~~Canada~~ toffee ~~lamb~~ mountain barber's pole sun ~~Africa~~ sea
drum paperclip treacle lava cola month triangle five blanket bed molten metal
cloud paper ~~France~~ pie maths subway pomp music fur piano keyboard pills
~~cow~~ wallet glue wrist ~~tiger~~ clown jam milk watch sand lake chilli pepper
stone ~~kitten~~ map quaver ~~baboon~~ stick carrot hitch ~~Paris~~ furnace broach ~~rat~~
diamond ~~Spain~~ paprika French flag guitar ~~goat~~ wallpaper paste square bag carrot
flipper horizon swimming ~~Brazil~~ ~~deer~~ brick hot tarmac ~~hamster~~ ~~antelope~~ balloon
conductor ~~kangaroo~~ nice radio ~~Cuba~~ underwear honey alphabet car curry
sergeant's chevrons

The following words are mentioned twice: sun, glue, diamond and carrot

Thinking Skills Exercise 22: Count the 'THEs' — Page 90

UNPICKING THE LOCK

Beethoven's secret revealed in his hair

THE life and work of Beethoven raise a number of intertwined questions. What made him so odd: clumsy; socially maladroit; ugly enough for a woman to whom he proposed to reject him for that alone; wildly irascible; increasingly in later life reclusive and paranoid? What caused him to lose his hearing before he was even 30? And – a question transcending all others – what was it that made him one of THE two or three greatest composers in THE history of music?

New evidence from THE United States suggests that some or possibly all of these things had something to do with lead. He was ill from his youth with a number of wretched conditions, especially dysentry. In 1802 he wrote to his brothers lamenting his fate and saying THE onset of deafness had brought him to THE brink of despair and close to ending his life. He was 31 – THE age at which Schubert died. He survived: but his problems grew worse. Now researchers in Chicago who have examined a lock of his hair believe he was suffering from lead poisoning. THE concentrations they found in THE hair were 100 times THE level of lead which is common today.

THE deaths of composers are often mysterious. Did Salieri murder Mozart? Did Tchaikovsky kill himself? There are plans to exhume Bellini, who may, some now think, have paid THE ultimate price for taking a woman away from her previous lover. At least in Beethoven's case murder is not alleged – yet. Drinking water, food or utensils are listed as possible culprits.

We know how much THE world would have lost had THE composer's despair overwhelmed him in 1802. What we cannot tell is whether THE music he wrote was shaped for better or worse by his malady; whether THE work of a healthier man might have been less profound than, say, THE last quartets or those final piano sonatas where Beethoven seems already beyond this world, somewhere nobler and more serene.

Total = 17

Thinking Skills Exercise 23: Count the 'OFs' — Page 91

An increase in the cost OF vital home care services used by the elderly, infirmed and disabled has been condemned by care groups and pensioners. The cost OF services such as meals on wheels, day centre provision and home helps is set to rise in April following a decision by the Berkshire social services committee meeting on Thursday 18 January.

Pensioners will also be hit by the level OF Disability Living Allowance paid back to the council for domiciliary services rising from 20 per cent to 50 per cent.

It is estimated the higher charges will net the council an additional £590,000 – £50,000 OF which has been earmarked for three new welfare benefit officers.

Jill Smith, who chairs Age Concern, said charges are spiraling 'out OF control'. She said: 'All these higher charges will affect the most vulnerable sets OF people in the community and it is just not on. This needs to be looked at more closely because very often it means that people will have to cut down on something else to meet the higher charges.'

Mrs Smith said that while daily charges were being increased by about 10p per day, the cost would be 'significant' over a period OF time. She said: 'The charge for meals on wheels adds up to 70p per week, and this is nearly half the cost OF a meal. Pensioners may go without one meal to make up for this.'

Mrs Smith also feels that many elderly people are reluctant – or unable – to complain, making them an easy target for higher charges. She added: 'Pensioners often do not stand up for themselves, and I feel that these sorts OF charges are spiraling out OF control.'

The changes, recommended in an Audit Commission document, were described in a report to councilors as the 'fairest way possible' OF increasing revenue. The report, by council officers, also said that the additional cash would be used to provide a greater number OF people with welfare benefits.

The report said: 'Local authorities have to balance concerns about charging vulnerable users with the ever-increasing need to fund the service. Managers have to reconcile the need to generate income with the potential negative effects OF charging, such as the anxiety charges can cause to users, and the cost OF administering the charges.'

Total = 14

Thinking Skills Exercise 24: Count the 'ANDs' — Page 92

BIRDS SET ALIGHT IN ART STUNT

Horrified shoppers AND young children saw pigeons being set alight as part of an arts festival. They have branded the bizarre ritual by a Spanish artist as 'sick', AND outraged officials of the Royal Society for the Protection of Birds fear some people will copy the stunt.

Controversial Jose Pallerno and his assistant used pigeons found dead on the streets for their act. But passers-by had no idea that was the case when they saw them blazing. Jose's act was part of the Manchester Biennial arts festival. When one angry shopper confronted him, he was told: 'I am burning my brothers.'

Jose said yesterday: 'I love pigeons very much AND it's not nice to see them dying on the street, squashed by cars. I wanted to do something related to the area, so I chose to work with pigeons, which symbolise the North AND the working classes.'

But Madeleine Pursley of the RSPB, said: 'We're horrified that anyone could justify this as an art form AND hope that no one else would entertain doing anything like this.'

This is not the first time that Jose Pallerno has been in the news; two years ago, as part of the Barcelona Arts Festival, he produced a work that stunned AND shocked art lovers everywhere. His piece, entitled Blood AND Guts, consisted of two hundred AND fifty metres of freshly slaughtered bulls' intestines, supported on six thousand matchsticks. Within hours of the exhibition opening the organisers had to remove the work because of the number of complaints about the smell!!

Total = 8

Thinking Skills Exercise 25: Keeping in mind — Page 93

7 + 2 = 9	2 – 1 = 1	5 + 4 = 9	5 + 2 = 7
2 + 3 = 5	M 5 + 8 =	7 * 3 = 4	7 – 6 = 1
4 – 2 = 2	9 – 6 = 3	8 – 5 = 3	5 * 3 = 8
6 + 2 = 8	3 * 4 = 7	4 * 3 = 7	3 – 2 = 1

5 * 2 = 3	2 + 7 = 9	7 * 2 = 5	6 * 2 = 8
6 – 4 = 2	3 * 2 = 1	M 5 + 5 =	5 – 4 = 1
M 7 + 4 =	M 6 + 2 =	1 – 1 = 0	M 9 + 3 =
9 – 7 = 2	3 – 3 = 0	2 + 3 = 5	1 + 2 = 3
M 8 – 3 =	4 + 2 = 6	M 4 – 3 =	3 + 4 = 7
5 * 1 = 6	6 + 6= 12	5 + 5 = 10	5 – 3 = 2
4 + 5 = 9	X 7 + 4 =	6 – 3 = 3	2 + 3 = 5
3 + 4 = 7	2 + 2=	M 6 + 6 =	9 * 4 = 5
X 6 + 3 =	9 * 6 =	3 + 3 = 6	X 4 – 3 =
6 – 4 =	1 – 1 =	X 2 + 1 =	2 + 6 =
2 * 5 =	3 + 3 =	1 + 2 =	8 * 8 =
1 + 4 =	7 + 1 =	8 + 9 =	7 – 2 =
Total = 53	Total = 39	Total = 52	Total = 48

Executive Skills Exercise 1: The main idea – birthday letter **Page 107**

1 (c) **2** D, D, D, M **3** (b)

Executive Skills Exercise 2: The main idea – holiday letter **Page 108**

1 (d) **2** D, M, D, D **3** (d)

Executive Skills Exercise 14: What are the emotions? **Page 120**

hostile **4** sorrow, tearful **12** very angry **2** sad **5** indifferent **1** sheepishly glad **9**
worried **10** happy **6** disgusted **8** sceptical **11** run-down, tired **7** shocked **3**

Executive Skills Exercise 18: Sentence sequencing **Page 127**

Correct order: C F A G E B D

Executive Skills Exercise 19: Planning courses **Page 128**

Which course would you enrol Jane on? Trampolining at Meadway, Saturday 10:00–11:00am, 5–8 years' beginners class.

Which course would you enrol Henry on? Diving at central pool, Saturday 9:00–9:30 am, 8+ years' improvers.

Executive Skills Exercise 24: Recognising emotions **Page 133**

Picture 1 – surprised
Picture 2 – furious
Picture 3 – worried
Picture 4 – thoughtful
Picture 5 – vain
Picture 6 – happy
Picture 7 – bored
Picture 8 – sad/tearful
Picture 9 – disgust

Awareness Skills Exercise 13: Social blunders **Page 168**

Story 1: Mary In order of significance: 1, 5, 3 *Story 2: Wayne* In order of significance: 3, 5

Adjustment Skills Exercise 23: Common misconceptions **Page 216**

Points that are true: 2, 4, 9, 11, 12 Points that are false: 1, 3, 5, 6, 7, 8, 10

Adjustment Exercise 30: Anger: ways of coping **Page 223**

1 I 2 G 3 K 4 A 5 H 6 B 7 J 8 C 9 D 10 F 11 E